W9-BRC-306

Current Clinical Strategies

Gynecology and Obstetrics

2004 Edition

New ACOG Treatment Guidelines

Paul D. Chan, M.D.

Susan M. Johnson, M.D.

Current Clinical Strategies Publishing

www.ccspublishing.com/ccs

Digital Book and Updates

Purchasers of this book may download the digital book and updates for Palm, Pocket PC, Windows and Macintosh. The digital book can be downloaded at the Current Clinical Strategies Publishing Internet site:

www.ccspublishing.com/ccs

Current Clinical Strategies Publishing
27071 Cabot Road
Laguna Hills, California 92653

Phone: 800-331-8227
Fax: 800-965-9420
Internet: www.ccspublishing.com/ccs
E-mail: info@ccspublishing.com

Printed in USA

ISBN 1929622-32-5

Contents

Surgical Documentation for Gynecology

Gynecologic Surgical History

Identifying Data. Age, gravida (number of pregnancies), para (number of deliveries).
Chief Compliant. Reason given by patient for seeking surgical care.
History of Present Illness (HPI). Describe the course of the patient's illness, including when it began, character of the symptoms; pain onset (gradual or rapid), character of pain (constant, intermittent, cramping, radiating); other factors associated with pain (urination, eating, strenuous activities); aggravating or relieving factors. Other related diseases; past diagnostic testing.
Obstetrical History. Past pregnancies, durations and outcomes, preterm deliveries, operative deliveries.
Gynecologic History: Last menstrual period, length of regular cycle.
Past Medical History (PMH). Past medical problems, previous surgeries, hospitalizations, diabetes, hypertension, asthma, heart disease.
Medications. Cardiac medications, oral contraceptives, estrogen.
Allergies. Penicillin, codeine.
Family History. Medical problems in relatives.
Social History. Alcohol, smoking, drug usage, occupation.
Review of Systems (ROS):
    General: Fever, fatigue, night sweats.
    HEENT: Headaches, masses, dizziness.
    Respiratory: Cough, sputum, dyspnea.
    Cardiovascular: Chest pain, extremity edema.
    Gastrointestinal: Vomiting, abdominal pain, melena (black tarry stools), hematochezia (bright red blood per rectum).
    Genitourinary: Dysuria, hematuria, discharge.
    Skin: Easy bruising, bleeding tendencies.

Gynecologic Physical Examination

General:
Vital Signs: Temperature, respirations, heart rate, blood pressure.
Eyes: Pupils equally round and react to light and accommodation (PERRLA); extraocular movements intact (EOMI).
Neck: Jugular venous distention (JVD), thyromegaly, masses, lymphadenopathy.
Chest: Equal expansion, rales, breath sounds.
Heart: Regular rate and rhythm (RRR), first and second heart sounds, murmurs.
Breast: Skin retractions, masses (mobile, fixed), erythema, axillary or supraclavicular node enlargement.
Abdomen: Scars, bowel sounds, masses, hepatosplenomegaly, guarding, rebound, costovertebral angle tenderness, hernias.
Genitourinary: Urethral discharge, uterus, adnexa, ovaries, cervix.
Extremities: Cyanosis, clubbing, edema.
Neurological: Mental status, strength, tendon reflexes, sensory testing.
Laboratory Evaluation: Electrolytes, glucose, liver function tests, INR/PTT, CBC with differential; X-rays, ECG (if >35 yrs or cardiovascular disease), urinalysis.
Assessment and Plan: Assign a number to each problem. Discuss each problem, and describe surgical plans for each numbered problem, including

preoperative testing, laboratory studies, medications, and antibiotics.

Discharge Summary

Patient's Name:
Chart Number:
Date of Admission:
Date of Discharge:
Admitting Diagnosis:
Discharge Diagnosis:
Name of Attending or Ward Service:
Surgical Procedures:
History and Physical Examination and Laboratory Data: Describe the course of the disease up to the time the patient came to the hospital, and describe the physical exam and laboratory data on admission.
Hospital Course: Describe the course of the patient's illness while in the hospital, including evaluation, treatment, outcome of treatment, and medications given.
Discharged Condition: Describe improvement or deterioration in condition.
Disposition: Describe the situation to which the patient will be discharged (home, nursing home).
Discharged Medications: List medications and instructions.
Discharged Instructions and Follow-up Care: Date of return for follow-up care at clinic; diet, exercise instructions.
Problem List: List all active and past problems.
Copies: Send copies to attending physician, clinic, consultants and referring physician.

Surgical Progress Note

Surgical progress notes are written in "SOAP" format.

Surgical Progress Note

Date/Time:
Post-operative Day Number:
Problem List: Antibiotic day number and hyperalimentation day number if applicable. List each surgical problem separately (eg, status-post appendectomy, hypokalemia).
Subjective: Describe how the patient feels in the patient's own words, and give observations about the patient. Indicate any new patient complaints, note the adequacy of pain relief, and passing of flatus or bowel movements. Type of food the patient is tolerating (eg, nothing, clear liquids, regular diet).
Objective:
    Vital Signs: Maximum temperature (T_{max}) over the past 24 hours. Current temperature, vital signs.
    Intake and Output: Volume of oral and intravenous fluids, volume of urine, stools, drains, and nasogastric output.
    Physical Exam:
        General appearance: Alert, ambulating.
        Heart: Regular rate and rhythm, no murmurs.
        Chest: Clear to auscultation.
        Abdomen: Bowel sounds present, soft, nontender.
        Wound Condition: Comment on the wound condition (eg, clean and dry, good granulation, serosanguinous drainage). Condition of dressings, purulent drainage, granulation tissue, erythema; condition of sutures, dehiscence. Amount and color of drainage
        Lab results: White count, hematocrit, and electrolytes, chest x-ray
Assessment and Plan: Evaluate each numbered problem separately. Note the patient's general condition (eg, improving), pertinent developments, and plans (eg, advance diet to regular, chest x-ray). For each numbered problem, discuss any additional orders and plans for discharge or transfer.

Procedure Note

A procedure note should be written in the chart when a procedure is performed. Procedure notes are brief operative notes.

Procedure Note

Date and time:
Procedure:
Indications:
Patient Consent: Document that the indications, risks and alternatives to the procedure were explained to the patient. Note that the patient was given the opportunity to ask questions and that the patient consented to the procedure in writing.
Lab tests: Electrolytes, INR, CBC
Anesthesia: Local with 2% lidocaine
Description of Procedure: Briefly describe the procedure, including sterile prep, anesthesia method, patient position, devices used, anatomic location of procedure, and outcome.
Complications and Estimated Blood Loss (EBL):
Disposition: Describe how the patient tolerated the procedure.
Specimens: Describe any specimens obtained and laboratory tests which were ordered.

Discharge Note

The discharge note should be written in the patient's chart prior to discharge.

Discharge Note

Date/time:
Diagnoses:
Treatment: Briefly describe treatment provided during hospitalization, including surgical procedures and antibiotic therapy.
Studies Performed: Electrocardiograms, CT scans.
Discharge Medications:
Follow-up Arrangements:

Postoperative Check

A postoperative check should be completed on the evening after surgery. This check is similar to a daily progress note.

Example Postoperative Check

Date/time:
Postoperative Check
Subjective: Note any patient complaints, and note the adequacy of pain relief.
Objective:
    General appearance:
    Vitals: Maximum temperature in the last 24 hours (T_{max}), current temperature, pulse, respiratory rate, blood pressure.
    Urine Output: If urine output is less than 30 cc per hour, more fluids should be infused if the patient is hypovolemic.
    Physical Exam:
    Chest and lungs:
    Abdomen:
    Wound Examination: The wound should be examined for excessive drainage or bleeding, skin necrosis, condition of drains.
    Drainage Volume: Note the volume and characteristics of drainage from Jackson-Pratt drain or other drains.
    Labs: Post-operative hematocrit value and other labs.
Assessment and Plan: Assess the patient's overall condition and status of wound. Comment on abnormal labs, and discuss treatment and discharge plans.

Total Abdominal Hysterectomy and Bilateral Salpingo-oophorectomy Operative Report

Preoperative Diagnosis: 45 year old female, gravida 3 para 3, with menometrorrhagia unresponsive to medical therapy.
Postoperative Diagnosis: Same as above
Operation: Total abdominal hysterectomy and bilateral salpingo-oophorectomy
Surgeon:
Assistant:
Anesthesia: General endotracheal
Findings At Surgery: Enlarged 10 x 12 cm uterus with multiple fibroids. Normal tubes and ovaries bilaterally. Frozen section revealed benign tissue. All specimens sent to pathology.
Description of Operative Procedure: After obtaining informed consent, the patient was taken to the operating room and placed in the supine position, given general anesthesia, and prepped and draped in sterile fashion.

A Pfannenstiel incision was made 2 cm above the symphysis pubis and extended sharply to the rectus fascia. The fascial incision was bilaterally incised with curved Mayo scissors, and the rectus sheath was separated superiorly and inferiorly by sharp and blunt dissection. The peritoneum was grasped between two Kelly clamps, elevated, and incised with a scalpel. The pelvis was examined with the findings noted above. A Balfour retractor was placed into the incision, and the bowel was packed away with moist laparotomy sponges. Two Kocher clamps were placed on the cornua of the uterus and used for retraction.

The round ligaments on both sides were clamped, sutured with #0 Vicryl, and transected. The anterior leaf of the broad ligament was incised along the bladder reflection to the midline from both sides, and the bladder was gently dissected off the lower uterine segment and cervix with a sponge stick.

The retroperitoneal space was opened and the ureters were identified bilaterally. The infundibulopelvic ligaments on both sides were then doubly clamped, transected, and doubly ligated with #O Vicryl. Excellent hemostasis was observed. The uterine arteries were skeletonized bilaterally, clamped with Heaney clamps, transected, and sutured with #O Vicryl. The uterosacral ligaments were clamped bilaterally, transected, and suture ligated in a similar fashion.

The cervix and uterus was amputated, and the vaginal cuff angles were closed with figure-of-eight stitches of #O Vicryl, and then were transfixed to the ipsilateral cardinal and uterosacral ligament. The vaginal cuff was closed with a series of interrupted #O Vicryl, figure-of-eight sutures. Excellent hemostasis was obtained.

The pelvis was copiously irrigated with warm normal saline, and all sponges and instruments were removed. The parietal peritoneum was closed with running #2-O Vicryl. The fascia was closed with running #O Vicryl. The skin was closed with stables. Sponge, lap, needle, and instrument counts were correct times two. The patient was taken to the recovery room, awake and in stable condition.

Estimated Blood Loss (EBL): 150 cc
Specimens: Uterus, tubes, and ovaries
Drains: Foley to gravity
Fluids: Urine output - 100 cc of clear urine
Complications: None
Disposition: The patient was taken to the recovery room in stable condition.

Vaginal Hysterectomy

Hysterectomy is the most common major operation performed on nonpregnant women. More than one-third of American women will undergo this procedure. The surgery may be approached abdominally, vaginally, or as a laparoscopically assisted vaginal procedure. The ratio of abdominal to vaginal hysterectomy is approximately 3:1.

I. **Indications for hysterectomy**
   A. Pelvic relaxation
   B. Leiomyomata
   C. Pelvic pain (eg, endometriosis)
   D. Abnormal uterine bleeding
   E. Adnexal mass
   F. Cervical intraepithelial neoplasia
   G. Endometrial hyperplasia
   H. Malignancy
   I. Pelvic relaxation is the most common indication and accounts for 45 percent of vaginal hysterectomies, while leiomyomata are the most common indication (40 percent) for the abdominal procedure.

II. **Route of hysterectomy**
   A. Vaginal hysterectomy is usually recommended for women with benign disease confined to the uterus when the uterine weight is estimated at less than 280 g. It is the preferred approach when pelvic floor repair is to be corrected concurrently.
   B. Contraindications to hysterectomy:
      1. Lack of uterine mobility
      2. Presence of an adnexal mass requiring removal
      3. Contracted bony pelvis
      4. Need to explore the upper abdomen
      5. Lack of surgical expertise
   C. Vaginal hysterectomy is associated with fewer complications, shorter length of hospitalization, and lower hospital charges than abdominal hysterectomy.

III. **Vaginal hysterectomy operative procedure**
   A. A prophylactic antibiotic agent (eg, cefazolin [Ancef] 1g IV) should be given as a single dose 30 minutes prior to the first incision for vaginal or abdominal hysterectomy.
   B. **Vaginal hysterectomy**
      1. The patient should be placed in the dorsal lithotomy position. When adequate anesthesia is obtained, a bimanual pelvic examination is performed to assess uterine mobility and descent and to confirm that no unsuspected adnexal disease is found. A final decision can then be made whether to proceed with a vaginal or abdominal approach.
      2. The patient is prepared and draped, and bladder catheter may be inserted. A weighted speculum is placed into the posterior vagina, a Deaver or right angle retractor is positioned anterior to the cervix, and then the anterior and posterior lips of the cervix are grasped with a single- or double-toothed tenaculum.
      3. Traction is placed on the cervix to expose the posterior vaginal mucosa. Using Mayo scissors, the posterior cul-de-sac is entered sharply, and the peritoneum identified. A figure-of-eight suture is then used to attach the peritoneum to the posterior vaginal mucosa.
      4. A Steiner-Anvard weighted speculum is inserted into the posterior cul-de-sac after this space is opened. The uterosacral ligaments are clamped, with the tip of the clamp incorporating the lower portion of the cardinal ligaments. The clamp is placed perpendicular to the uterine axis, and the pedicle cut so that there is 0.5 cm of tissue distal to the clamp. A transfixion suture is then placed at the tip of the clamp. Once ligated, the uterosacral ligaments are transfixed to the posterior lateral vaginal mucosa. This suture is held with a hemostat.
      5. Downward traction is placed on the cervix to provide countertraction for the vaginal mucosa and the anterior vaginal mucosa is incised at the level of the cervicovaginal junction. The bladder is advanced upward using an open, moistened gauze sponge. At this point, the vesicovaginal peritoneal reflection is usually identified and can be entered sharply using scissors. A Deaver or Heaney retractor is placed in the midline to keep the bladder out of the operative field. Blunt or sharp advancement of the bladder should precede each clamp placement until the vesicovaginal space is entered.
      6. The cardinal ligaments are identified, clamped, cut, and suture ligated. The bladder is advanced out of the operative field using blunt dissection technique. The uterine vessels are clamped to incorporate the anterior and posterior leaves of the visceral peritoneum.
      7. The anterior peritoneal fold is now visualized, and the anterior cul-de-sac can be entered. The peritoneal reflection is grasped with smooth forceps, tented, and opened with scissors with the tips pointed toward the uterus. A Heaney or Deaver retractor is placed into this space to protect the bladder.
      8. The uterine fundus is delivered posteriorly by placing a tenaculum on the uterine fundus in successive bites. An index finger is used to identify the utero-ovarian ligament and aid in clamp placement. The remainder of the utero-ovarian ligaments are clamped and cut. The pedicles are double-ligated first with a suture tie and followed by a suture ligature medial to the first tie.
IV. **Discharge instructions**
   A. The woman is encouraged to resume her normal daily activities as quickly as is comfortable. Walking and stair climbing are encouraged; tub baths or showers are permissible.
   B. The patient should avoid lifting over 20 lb of weight for four to six weeks after surgery to minimize stress on the healing fascia. Vaginal intercourse is discouraged during this period. Driving should be avoided until full mobility returns and narcotic analgesia is no longer required.

Endometrial Sampling and Dilation and Curettage

The endometrial cavity is frequently evaluated because of abnormal uterine bleeding, pelvic pain, infertility, or pregnancy complications. The most common diagnostic indications for obtaining endometrial tissue include abnormal uterine bleeding, postmenopausal bleeding, endometrial dating, endometrial cells on Papanicolaou smear, and follow-up of women undergoing medical therapy for endometrial hyperplasia.

I. Endometrial biopsy

A. The office endometrial biopsy offers a number of advantages to D&C because it can be done with minimal to no cervical dilation, anesthesia is not required, and the cost is approximately one-tenth of a hospital D&C.

B. Numerous studies have shown that the endometrium is adequately sampled with these techniques.

C. Pipelle endometrial sampling device is the most popular method for sampling the endometrial lining. The device is constructed of flexible polypropylene with an outer sheath measuring 3.1 mm in diameter.

D. The device is placed in the uterus through an undilated cervix. The piston is fully withdrawn to create suction and, while the device is rotated 360 degrees, the distal port is brought from the fundus to the internal os to withdraw a sample. The device is removed and the distal aspect of the instrument is severed, allowing for the expulsion of the sample into form-alin.

E. The detection rates for endometrial cancer by Pipelle in postmenopausal and premenopausal women are 99.6 and 91 percent, respectively.

F. D&C should be considered when the endometrial biopsy is nondiagnostic, but a high suspicion of cancer remains (eg, hyperplasia with atypia, presence of necrosis, or pyometra).

II. Dilation and curettage

A. Dilation and curettage is performed as either a diagnostic or therapeutic procedure. Indications for diagnostic D&C include:

    1. A nondiagnostic office biopsy in women who are at high risk of endometrial carcinoma.

    2. Insufficient tissue for analysis on office biopsy.

    3. Cervical stenosis prevents the completion of an office biopsy.

B. Diagnostic D&Cs are usually performed with hysteroscopy to obtain a visual image of the endometrial cavity, exclude focal disease, and prevent missing unsuspected polyps.

C. Examination under anesthesia. After anesthesia has been administered, the size, shape, and position of the uterus are noted, with particular attention to the axis of the cervix and flexion of the fundus. The size, shape, and consistency of the adnexa are determined. The perineum, vagina, and cervix are then prepared with an aseptic solution and vaginal retractors are inserted into the vagina.

D. Operative technique. A D&C is performed with the woman in the dorsal lithotomy position.

    1. Endocervical curettage (ECC) is performed before dilation of the cervix. A Kevorkian-Younge curette is introduced into the cervical canal up to the internal os. Curetting of all four quadrants of the canal should be conducted and the specimen placed on a Telfa pad.

    2. Sounding and dilation. Traction is applied to align the axis of the cervix and the uterine canal. The uterus should be sounded to document the size and confirm the position. The sound should be held between the thumb and the index finger to avoid excessive pressure.

    3. Cervical dilation is then performed. The dilator is grasped in the middle of the instrument with the thumb and index finger. The cervix is gradually dilated beginning with the #13 French Pratt dilator. The dilator should be inserted through the internal os, without excessively entering the uterine cavity.

4. **Sharp curettage** is performed systematically beginning at the fundus and applying even pressure on the endometrial surface along the entire length of the uterus to the internal cervical os. The endometrial tissue is placed on a Telfa pad placed in the vagina. Moving around the uterus in a systematic fashion, the entire surface of the endometrium is sampled. The curettage procedure is completed when the "uterine cry" (grittiness to palpation) is appreciated on all surfaces of the uterus. Curettage is followed by blind extraction with Randall polyp forceps to improve the rate of detection of polyps.

General Gynecology

Management of the Abnormal Papanicolaou Smear

The Papanicolaou smear is a screening test for abnormalities that increases the risk of cervical cancer. Treatment decisions are based upon the results of colposcopically directed biopsies of the cervix. Papanicolaou smear reports are classified using the Bethesda System, which was revised in 2001.

I. Pap Smear Report

Bethesda 2001 Pap Smear Report

Interpretation Result
Negative for intraepithelial lesion or malignancy (when there is no cellular evidence of neoplasia, state this in the General Categorization above and/or in the Interpretation/Result section of the report, whether there are organisms or other non-neoplastic findings)
Infection (Trichomonas vaginalis, Candida spp., shift in flora suggestive of bacterial vaginosis, Actinomyces spp., cellular changes consistent with Herpes simplex virus)
Other Non-neoplastic Findings (Optional to report; list not inclusive):
    Reactive cellular changes associated with inflammation (includes typical repair) radiation, intrauterine contraceptive device (IUD)
    Glandular cells status post-hysterectomy
    Atrophy
Other
    Endometrial cells (in a woman ≥40 years of age) (specify if "negative for squamous intraepithelial lesion")
Epithelial Cell Abnormalities
  Squamous Cell
    Atypical squamous cells
      -of undetermined significance (ASC-US)
      -cannot exclude HSIL (ASC-H)
    Low-grade squamous intraepithelial lesion (LSIL) encompassing: HPV/mild dysplasia/CIN 1
    High-grade squamous intraepithelial lesion (HSIL) encompassing: moderate and severe dysplasia, CIS/CIN 2 and CIN 3 with features suspicious for invasion (if invasion is suspected)
    Squamous cell carcinoma
  Glandular Cell
    Atypical
      -Endocervical cells (not otherwise specified or specify in comments)
      -Glandular Cell (not otherwise specified or specify in comments)
      -Endometrial cells (not otherwise specified or specify in comments)
      -Glandular cells (not otherwise specified or specify in comments)
    Atypical
      -Endocervical cells, favor neoplastic
      -Glandular cells, favor neoplastic
    Endocervical adenocarcinoma in situ
    Adenocarcinoma (endocervical, endometrial, extrauterine, not otherwise specified (not otherwise specified)
Other Malignant Neoplasms (specify)

II. Screening for cervical cancer

A. Regular Pap smears are recommended for all women who are or have been sexually active and who have a cervix.

B. Testing should begin when the woman first engages in sexual intercourse. Adolescents whose sexual history is thought to be unreliable should be presumed to be sexually active at age 18.

C. Pap smears should be performed at least every 1 to 3 years. Testing is usually discontinued after age 65 in women who have had regular normal screening tests. Women who have had a hysterectomy, including removal of the cervix for reasons other than cervical cancer or its precursors, do not require Pap testing.

III. **Techniques used in evaluation of the abnormal pap smear**
   A. **Colposcopy** allows examination of the lower genital tract to identify epithelial changes. Abnormal areas should be targeted for biopsy to determine a pathologic diagnosis.
   B. **Human papillomavirus testing**
      1. HPV infection is the leading etiologic agent in the development of premalignant and malignant lower genital tract disease. Premenopausal women who test positive for certain types of HPV are at higher risk of cervical dysplasia (HPV positive), while those who are HPV negative or have types of HPV DNA of low oncogenic potential are at low risk.
      2. The most commonly used HPV test is the Hybrid Capture II HPV DNA Assay (HC II), which tests for high-risk HPV types 16, 18, 31, 33, 35, 39, 45, 51, 52, 56, 58, 59, and 68. High-risk HPV types 16 and 18 are the viruses most frequently isolated in cervical cancer tissue.

IV. **Atypical squamous cells**
   A. **Atypical squamous cells of undetermined significance (ASCUS)** is further divided into ASC-US, which are qualified as "of undetermined significance," and ASC-H, in which a high-grade squamous intraepithelial lesion (HSIL) cannot be excluded.
   B. ASC requires further evaluation. This cytologic diagnosis is common and frequently associated with spontaneously resolving, self-limited disease. However, 5 to 17 percent of patients with ASC and 24 to 94 percent of those with ASC-H will have CIN II or III at biopsy.
   C. **Women with ASC-US**
      1. **Management of minimally abnormal cervical cytology smears (ASC-US):**
         a. If liquid-based cytology is used, reflex testing for HPV should be performed, alternatively cocollection for HPV DNA testing can be done at the time of a conventional cervical cytology smear.
         b. Colposcopy should be performed if human papillomavirus testing is positive. Thirty to 60 percent of women with ASC will test positive for high-risk HPV types and require immediate colposcopy.
      2. Patients with a positive high-risk type HPV DNA test should be evaluated by colposcopy; those with a negative test may be triaged to repeat cytologic evaluation in 12 months. Management of women who test positive for high-risk HPV types, but have no CIN consists of either 1) cytological testing repeated in six and 12 months with colposcopic evaluation of ASC-US or greater or 2) HPV testing repeated in 12 months with colposcopy if HPV results are positive.

V. **Special circumstances**
   A. **When an infectious organism is identified**, the patient should be contacted to determine if she is symptomatic. Antibiotic therapy is indicated for symptomatic infection.
   B. **Reactive changes due to inflammation** are usually not associated with an organism on the Pap smear. The Pap smear does not need to be repeated unless the patient is HIV positive, in which case it should be repeated in four to six months.
   C. **Atrophic epithelium** is a normal finding in postmenopausal women.
      1. Administration of estrogen causes atypical atrophic, but not dysplastic, epithelium to mature into normal squamous epithelium.
      2. Hormonal therapy given for vaginal atrophy should be followed by repeat cervical cytology one week after completing treatment. If negative, cytology should be repeated again in four to six months. If both tests are negative, the woman can return to routine screening intervals, but if either test is positive for ASC-US or greater, she should be evaluated with colposcopy.
   D. **Immunosuppressed women**, including all women who are HIV positive, with ASC-US should be referred for immediate colposcopy, instead of HPV testing.

E. **ASC-US with absence of CIN on biopsy**. If colposcopic examination does not show CIN, then follow-up cytological testing should be performed in 12 months.

F. **ASC-US with biopsy proven CIN.** Since spontaneous regression is observed in approximately 60 percent of CIN I, expectant management with serial cytologic smears at three to four month intervals is reasonable for the reliable patient.

G. **Women with ASC-H.** All women with ASC-H on cytological examination should receive colposcopy. If repeat of cytology confirms ASC-H but biopsy is negative for CIN, follow-up cytology in six and 12 months or HPV DNA testing in 12 months is recommended. Colposcopy should be repeated for ASC or greater on cytology or a positive test for high risk HPV DNA. Biopsy proven CIN is treated, as appropriate.

VI. **Low- and high-grade intraepithelial neoplasia**

A. **Low-grade squamous intraepithelial lesions (LSIL)** may also be referred to as CIN I or mild dysplasia. Immediate referral for colposcopy is the recommended management for LSIL. Endocervical sampling should be done in nonpregnant women in whom the transformation zone cannot be fully visualized or a lesion extends into the endocervical canal. Endocervical sampling also should be done in nonpregnant women when no lesion is identified on colposcopy.

1. If no CIN is identified following satisfactory or unsatisfactory colposcopy and biopsies, then options for follow-up include either:
   a. Repeat cytology testing at six and 12 months, or
   b. HPV DNA testing at 12 months
2. Referral for repeat colposcopy is required if cytology yields ASC or greater or HPV DNA is positive for a high-risk type.
3. Women with histologically confirmed CIN I LSIL may be treated with ablation or excision or followed with serial cytologic smears every three to six months if the entire lesion and limits of the transformation zone are completely visualized. LSIL confined to the endocervical canal may be followed with repeat smears obtained with a cytobrush and with ECC.
4. **Postmenopausal women.** Postmenopausal women may be managed by serial cytology at six and 12 months or HPV DNA testing at 12 months with referral to colposcopy for positive results. Women with atrophy are treated with intravaginal estrogen followed by repeat cytology seven days after completion of therapy, with referral to colposcopy if an abnormality persists. If repeat cytology is normal, then another cytology test should be obtained in four to six months. The woman can return to routine surveillance if both tests are normal, but should be referred for colposcopy if either test is positive.
5. **Adolescents.** Initial colposcopy may be deferred in adolescents. Instead, they may be managed with serial cytology at six and 12 months or HPV DNA testing at 12 months with referral to colposcopy for positive results.
6. **Pregnant women.** Colposcopy should be performed, with biopsy and endocervical curettage performed for any lesion suspicious for HSIL or more severe disease.

B. **High-grade squamous intraepithelial lesions**

1. A high-grade squamous intraepithelial lesion (HSIL) may also be referred to as CIN II or III, severe dysplasia, or carcinoma in situ (CIS). One to two percent of women with HSIL on a cytologic smear have invasive cancer at the time of further evaluation and 20 percent of women with biopsy-proven CIS will develop an invasive cancer if left untreated. All women with HSIL should be referred for colposcopy and endocervical sampling.

C. **Follow-up evaluation.** Pap smears are recommended every three to four months for the first year after treatment for dysplasia. Women with cervical dysplasia present at the LEEP or cone margin or in the concomitant ECC also need a follow-up colposcopy with endocervical curettage every six months for one year. Routine surveillance can be resumed if there is no recurrence after the first year. Surveillance consists of Pap smears on a yearly basis for most women, and on a twice-yearly basis for high-risk women (ie, HIV positive).

VII. Abnormal glandular cells
    A. A report of atypical glandular cells (AGC) indicates the presence of glandular cells that could be coming from the endocervical or endometrial region. The Bethesda 2001 system classifies AGC into two subcategories:
        1. AGC endocervical, endometrial, or not otherwise specified (NOS)
        2. AGC favor neoplasia, endocervical or NOS
    B. Additional categories for glandular cell abnormalities are:
        1. Endocervical adenocarcinoma in situ (AIS)
        2. Adenocarcinoma
    C. **Evaluation of AGC or AIS on cervical cytology:** These women should be referred for colposcopy and sampling of the endocervical canal. Women over age 35 and younger women with AGC and unexplained vaginal bleeding also need an endometrial biopsy. Women with only atypical endometrial cells on cytology can be initially evaluated with endometrial biopsy.
    D. **Endometrial cells in women ≥40 years of age:** Endometrial biopsy should be performed.

References: See page 166.

Cervical Intraepithelial Neoplasia

Cervical intraepithelial neoplasia refers to a preinvasive precursor of cervical cancer which can be easily detected and treated. Over 50,000 new cases of carcinoma in situ are diagnosed annually. The prevalence of CIN varies from as low as 1.05 percent in family planning or general gynecology clinics to as high as 13.7 percent in sexually transmitted disease clinics.

I. Nomenclature
    A. Cervical intraepithelial neoplasia (CIN) divides the epithelial thickness into thirds.
        1. CIN I refers cellular dysplasia confined to the basal third of the epithelium.
        2. CIN II refers to lesions confined to the basal two-thirds of the epithelium.
        3. CIN III refers to cellular dysplasia encompassing greater than two-thirds of the epithelial thickness, including full-thickness lesions previously termed CIS.
    B. Histologically evaluated lesions are graded using the CIN nomenclature, while cytologic smears are classified according to the Bethesda system.

II. Epidemiology and pathogenesis
    A. CIN is typically detected at an age 10 to 15 years younger than that reported for invasive cervical carcinoma. The diagnosis of CIN is usually made in women in their 20s, carcinoma in situ is diagnosed in women 25 to 35 years of age, and invasive cancer after the age of 40.
    B. **Human papillomavirus** (HPV) infection is the leading cause of premalignant and malignant lower genital tract disease. HPV is found in 70-78 percent of patients with CIN I and in 83-89 percent of CIN II/III. Risk factors for CIN include sexual activity at an early age, history of sexually transmitted diseases, multiple sexual partners, or sexual activity with promiscuous men. Other risk factors include cigarette smoking, multiparity, and immunodeficiency.

III. Diagnosis
    A. Women are typically screened for CIN by cervical cytology (eg, direct Papanicolaou smear, ThinPrep).
    B. Abnormal cytology results should be further evaluated. Evaluation of the cervix following abnormal cytology results includes visual inspection, repeat cytology, colposcopy, directed biopsy, and endocervical curettage.

IV. **Colposcopy**
   A. Colposcopy is the primary technique for evaluation of abnormal cytology. Abnormal areas of the epithelium turn white following the application of dilute acetic acid. Capillaries may be identified within the abnormal epithelium. High-grade lesions tend to have a coarser vessel pattern and larger intercapillary distance. Abnormal areas can be targeted for biopsy.
   B. **Indications for colposcopy:**
      1. Abnormal cervical cytology smear
      2. Abnormal findings on adjunctive screening techniques, such as HPV testing or cervicography
      3. Clinically abnormal or suspicious looking cervix
      4. Unexplained intermenstrual or postcoital bleeding
      5. Vulvar or vaginal neoplasia
   C. **Technique**
      1. **A repeat cervical cytology smear** is performed prior to colposcopy if more than three months have elapsed since the index smear.
      2. **The cervix is cleansed and moistened** with normal saline and visualized through the colposcope. White lesions are recorded as leukoplakia on a diagram of the cervix.
      3. **A green-filter examination** is performed to enhance the vascular architecture and detect atypical vessels.
      4. **Acetic acid 3-5%** is applied with cotton swabs for 30 seconds to stain the cervix. Areas of acetowhite epithelium and abnormal vascular patterns are noted.
      5. If the entire transformation zone and squamocolumnar junction can be visualized, the colposcopy is satisfactory; otherwise, it is unsatisfactory.
      6. **Biopsies** are obtained from the areas with the most severe abnormalities, including leukoplakia, atypical vessels, acetowhite epithelium, punctations, and mosaicism. Bleeding can be controlled with Monsel's solution or silver nitrate application.
      7. **Endocervical curettage** should be performed.
V. **Management of cervical intraepithelial neoplasia**
   A. **Women with atypical squamous cells (ASC) or low-grade squamous intraepithelial lesions (LGSIL or LSIL)**
      1. **Minimally abnormal cervical cytology.** Atypical squamous cells (ASC) or low-grade squamous intraepithelial lesions (LGSIL or LSIL) is common and frequently associated with spontaneously resolving, self-limited disease. However, 9 to 19 percent of patients with ASC or LGSIL will have CIN II or III at colposcopy.
      2. Atypical squamous cells requires further evaluation and treatment may be initiated if there is biopsy proven dysplasia.
   B. **LSIL/CIN I**
      1. Since spontaneous regression is observed in more than 60 percent of biopsy-confirmed CIN I (mild dysplasia), expectant management with serial cytologic smears at three to four month intervals may be the preferable management for the reliable patient. Repeat colposcopy is required for any abnormal cervical cytology smear. A lesion that persists after 1 to 2 years or any progression during the follow-up period suggests the need for treatment.
      2. Some women may elect to have ablation or excision of the lesion to relieve anxiety.
   C. **HSIL**
      1. Women with high grade squamous intraepithelial lesions (HGSIL or HSIL) on cervical cytology smear are evaluated by colposcopy, endocervical curettage (ECC), and directed biopsies. Treatment may include procedures that ablate the abnormal tissue and do not produce a specimen for additional histologic evaluation or procedures that excise the area of abnormality, allowing for further histologic study. An assessment has to be made as to whether a patient qualifies for ablative therapy or if she requires conization for excision and further diagnostic evaluation.

2. **Requirements for ablative treatment:**
    a. Accurate histologic diagnosis/no discrepancy between Pap/colpo-scopy/histology
    b. No evidence of microinvasion/invasion
    c. No evidence of glandular lesion (adenocarcinoma in situ or invasive adenocarcinoma)
    d. Satisfactory colposcopy (the transformation zone is fully visualized)
    e. The lesion is limited to the ectocervix and seen in its entirety
    f. There is no evidence of endocervical involvement as determined by colposcopy/ECC
3. The most commonly used ablative treatment techniques are cryo-therapy and laser ablation.
4. **Indications for conization are:**
    a. Suspected microinvasion
    b. Unsatisfactory colposcopy (the transformation zone is not fully visualized)
    c. Lesion extending into endocervical canal
    d. ECC revealing dysplasia
    e. Lack of correlation between the Pap smear and colposcopy/biop-sies
    f. Suspected adenocarcinoma in situ
    g. Colposcopist unable to rule out invasive disease
5. Excisional treatment can be performed by cold knife conization using a scalpel, laser conization, or the loop electrosurgical excision procedure (LEEP), also called large loop excision of the transformation zone (LLETZ).

D. **Specific therapeutic techniques**
  1. **Common techniques for treatment of CIN:**
      a. Cryotherapy (nitrous oxide or carbon dioxide)
      b. Loop electrosurgical excision procedure (LEEP, LLETZ).
      c. Carbon dioxide (CO_2) laser ablation
      d. Excisional (cold knife) conization
      e. Carbon dioxide laser cone excision
  2. The techniques are of equal efficacy, averaging approximately 90 percent efficacy.
  3. **Cryotherapy**
      a. Cryotherapy consists of the application of a super-cooled probe directly to the cervical lesion using two cooling and thawing cycles. The probe must be able to cover the entire lesion and the lesion cannot extend into the endocervical canal.
      b. The multiple cycle freeze-thaw-freeze technique should be used, and the blanching should extend at least 7 to 8 mm beyond the edge of the cryo-probe to reach the full depth of the cervical crypts. Mild cramping accompanies the procedure.
      c. The advantages of this approach include low cost and a low complication rate. Disadvantages are a copious vaginal discharge lasting for weeks and a lack of tissue for histology.
  4. **Loop electrosurgical excision procedure**
      a. The loop electrosurgical excision procedure (LEEP or LLETZ) has become the approach of choice for treating CIN II and III because of its ease of use, low cost, and high rate of success. It can be performed in the office using local anesthesia.
      b. The procedure uses a wire loop through which an electrical current is passed. The transformation zone and lesion are excised to a variable depth, which should be at least 8 mm, and extending 4 to 5 mm beyond the lesion. An additional endocervical specimen is frequently removed to allow histologic evaluation.

E. **Adenocarcinoma in situ**
  1. The Bethesda 2001 system classifies glandular cell abnormalities into four subcategories:
      a. Atypical glandular cells endocervical, endometrial, or not otherwise specified (NOS)

   b. Atypical glandular cells favor neoplastic, endocervical or endometrial
   c. Endocervical adenocarcinoma in situ (AIS)
   d. Adenocarcinoma
2. The categories AGC favor neoplasia and AIS have a somewhat higher likelihood of being associated with significant disease than AGC NOS.
3. AIS is a precursor of adenocarcinoma of the cervix. The diagnosis is based upon histology. The lesion may be located high in the endocervical canal.
4. The incidence of residual AIS or invasive adenocarcinoma following conization for AIS is high. If conization margins are positive, repeat conization should be performed in patients who wish to maintain fertility. If fertility is not desired, hysterectomy should be performed as the definitive therapeutic intervention.

F. Follow-up
   1. Patients with positive margins after LEEP or cold knife conization are at increased risk for residual disease.
   2. Careful clinical follow-up with cytology and colposcopy/biopsy (when indicated) in women with positive margins, instead of immediate retreatment, is appropriate in patients who are compliant with frequent monitoring. Cytologic assessment should be continued at three month intervals until normal for one year after therapy and yearly thereafter.

References: See page 166.

Contraception

Approximately 31 percent of births are unintended; about 22 percent were "mistimed," while 9 percent were "unwanted."

I. Sterilization
   A. Sterilization is the most common and effective form of contraception. While tubal ligation and vasectomy may be reversible, these procedures should be considered permanent.
   B. **Essure microinsert sterilization device** is a permanent, hysteroscopic, tubal sterilization device which is 99.9 percent effective. The coil-like device is inserted in the office under local anesthesia into the fallopian tubes where it is incorporated by tissue. After placement, women use alternative contraception for three months, after which hysterosalpingography is performed to assure correct placement. Postoperative discomfort is minimal.
   C. **Tubal ligation** is usually performed as a laparoscopic procedure in outpatients or in postpartum women in the hospital. The techniques used are unipolar or bipolar coagulation, silicone rubber band or spring clip application, and partial salpingectomy.
   D. **Vasectomy** (ligation of the vas deferens) can be performed in the office under local anesthesia. A semen analysis should be done three to six months after the procedure to confirm azoospermia.

II. Oral contraceptives
   A. Combined (estrogen-progestin) oral contraceptives are reliable, and they have noncontraceptive benefits, which include reduction in dysmenorrhea, iron deficiency, ovarian cancer, endometrial cancer.

Combination Oral Contraceptives

Drug	Progestin, mg	Estrogen
Monophasic combinations		
Ortho-Novum 1 /35 21, 28	Norethindrone (1)	Ethinyl estradiol (35)
Ovcon 35 21, 28	Norethindrone (0.4)	Ethinyl estradiol (35)
Brevicon 21, 28	Norethindrone (0.5)	Ethinyl estradiol (35)
Modicon 28	Norethindrone (0.5)	Ethinyl estradiol (35)
Necon 0.5/35E 21, 28	Norethindrone (0.5)	Ethinyl estradiol (35)
Nortrel 0.5/35 28	Norethindrone (0.5)	Ethinyl estradiol (35)
Necon 1 /35 21, 28	Norethindrone (1)	Ethinyl estradiol (35)
Norinyl 1 /35 21, 28	Norethindrone (1)	Ethinyl estradiol (35)
Nortrel 1 /35 21, 28	Norethindrone (1)	Ethinyl estradiol (35)
Loestrin 1 /20 21, 28	Norethindrone acetate (1)	Ethinyl estradiol (20)
Microgestin 1 /20 28	Norethindrone acetate (1)	Ethinyl estradiol (20)
Loestrin 1.5/30 21, 28	Norethindrone acetate (1.5)	Ethinyl estradiol (30)
Microgestin 1.5/30 28	Norethindrone acetate (1.5)	Ethinyl estradiol (30)
Alesse 21, 28	Levonorgestrel (0.1)	Ethinyl estradiol (20)
Aviane 21, 28	Levonorgestrel (0.1)	Ethinyl estradiol (20)
Lessina 28	Levonorgestrel (0.1)	Ethinyl estradiol (20)
Levlite 28	Levonorgestrel (0.1)	Ethinyl estradiol (20)
Necon 1/50 21, 28	Norethindrone (1)	Mestranol (50)
Norinyl 1150 21, 28	Norethindrone (1)	Mestranol (50)
Ortho-Novum 1/50 28	Norethindrone (1)	Mestranol (50)
Ovcon 50 28	Norethindrone (1)	Ethinyl estradiol (50)
Cyclessa 28	Desogestrel (0.1)	Ethinyl estradiol (25)
Apri 28	Desogestrel (0.15)	Ethinyl estradiol (30)
Desogen 28	Desogestrel (0.15)	Ethinyl estradiol (30)
Ortho-Cept 21, 28	Desogestrel (0.15)	Ethinyl estradiol (30)

Drug	Progestin, mg	Estrogen
Yasmin 28	Drospirenone (3)	Ethinyl estradiol (30)
Demulen 1 /35 21, 28	Ethynodiol diacetate (1)	Ethinyl estradiol (35)
Zovia 1 /35 21, 28	Ethynodiol diacetate (1)	Ethinyl estradiol (35)
Demulen 1/50 21, 28	Ethynodiol diacetate (1)	Ethinyl estradiol (50)
Zovia 1 /50 21, 28	Ethynodiol diacetate (1)	Ethinyl estradiol (50)
Levlen 21, 28	Levonorgestrel (0.15)	Ethinyl estradiol (30)
Levora 21, 28	Levonorgestrel (0.15)	Ethinyl estradiol (30)
Nordette 21, 28	Levonorgestrel (0.15)	Ethinyl estradiol (30)
Ortho-Cyclen 21, 28	Norgestimate (0.25)	Ethinyl estradiol (35)
Lo/Ovral 21, 28	Norgestrel (0.3)	Ethinyl estradiol (30)
Low-Ogestrel 21, 28	Norgestrel (0.3)	Ethinyl estradiol (30)
Ogestrel 28	Norgestrel (0.5)	Ethinyl estradiol (50)
Ovral 21, 28	Norgestrel (0.5)	Ethinyl estradiol (50)
Multiphasic Combinations		
Kariva 28	Desogestrel (0.15)	Ethinyl estradiol (20, 0, 10)
Mircette 28	Desogestrel (0.15)	Ethinyl estradiol (20, 0, 10)
Tri-Levlen 21, 28	Levonorgestrel (0.05, 0.075, 0.125)	Ethinyl estradiol (30, 40, 30)
Triphasil 21, 28	Levonorgestrel (0.05, 0.075, 0.125)	Ethinyl estradiol (30, 40, 30)
Trivora 28	Levonorgestrel (0.05, 0.075, 0.125)	Ethinyl estradiol (30, 40, 30)
Necon 10/11 21, 28	Norethindrone (0.5, 1)	Ethinyl estradiol (35)
Ortho-Novum 10/11 28	Norethindrone (0.5, 1)	Ethinyl estradiol (35)
Ortho-Novum 7/7/7 21, 28	Norethindrone (0.5, 0.75, 1)	Ethinyl estradiol (35)
Tri-Norinyl 21, 28	Norethindrone (0.5, 1, 0.5)	Ethinyl estradiol (35)
Estrostep 28	Norethindrone acetate (1)	Ethinyl estradiol (20, 30, 35)
Ortho Tri-Cyclen 21, 28	Norgestimate (0.18, 0.215, 0.25)	Ethinyl estradiol (35)

B. Pharmacology
  1. Ethinyl estradiol is the estrogen in virtually all OCs.
  2. Commonly used progestins include norethindrone, norethindrone acetate, and levonorgestrel. Ethynodiol diacetate is a progestin, which also has significant estrogenic activity. New progestins have been developed with less androgenic activity; however, these agents may be associated with deep vein thrombosis.
C. Mechanisms of action
  1. The most important mechanism of action is estrogen-induced inhibition of the midcycle surge of gonadotropin secretion, so that ovulation does not occur.
  2. Another potential mechanism of contraceptive action is suppression of gonadotropin secretion during the follicular phase of the cycle, thereby preventing follicular maturation.
  3. Progestin-related mechanisms also may contribute to the contraceptive effect. These include rendering the endometrium is less suitable for implantation and making the cervical mucus less permeable to penetration by sperm.
D. Contraindications
  1. **Absolute contraindications to OCs:**
     a. Previous thromboembolic event or stroke
     b. History of an estrogen-dependent tumor
     c. Active liver disease
     d. Pregnancy
     e. Undiagnosed abnormal uterine bleeding
     f. Hypertriglyceridemia
     g. Women over age 35 years who smoke heavily (greater than 15 cigarettes per day)
  2. **Screening requirements.** Hormonal contraception can be safely provided after a careful medical history and blood pressure measurement. Pap smears are not required before a prescription for OCs.
E. Efficacy. When taken properly, OCs are a very effective form of contraception. The actual failure rate is 2 to 3 percent due primarily to missed pills or failure to resume therapy after the seven-day pill-free interval.

Noncontraceptive Benefits of Oral Contraceptive Pills	
Dysmenorrhea	Functional ovarian cysts
Mittelschmerz	Benign breast cysts
Metrorrhagia	Ectopic pregnancy
Premenstrual syndrome	Acne
Hirsutism	Endometriosis
Ovarian and endometrial cancer	

F. Drug interactions. The metabolism of OCs is accelerated by phenobarbital, phenytoin and rifampin. The contraceptive efficacy of an OC is likely to be decreased in women taking these drugs. Other antibiotics (with the exception of rifampin) do not affect the pharmacokinetics of ethinyl estradiol.
G. Preparations
  1. There are two types of oral contraceptive pills: combination pills that contain both estrogen and progestin, and the progestin-only pill ("minipill"). Progestin-only pills, which are associated with more breakthrough bleeding than combination pills, are rarely prescribed except in lactating women. Combination pills are packaged in 21-day or 28-day cycles. The last seven pills of a 28-day pack are placebo pills.
  2. Monophasic combination pills contain the same dose of estrogen and progestin in each of the 21 hormonally active pills. Current pills contain on average 30 to 35 μg. Pills containing less than 50 μg of ethinyl estradiol are "low-dose" pills.

3. **20 µg preparations.** Several preparations containing only 20 µg of ethinyl estradiol are now available (Lo-Estrin 1/20, Mircette, Alesse, Aviane). These are often used for perimenopausal women who want contraception with the lowest estrogen dose possible. These preparations provide enough estrogen to relieve vasomotor flashes. Perimenopausal women often experience hot flashes and premenstrual mood disturbances during the seven-day pill-free interval. Mircette, contains 10 µg of ethinyl estradiol on five of the seven "placebo" days, which reduces flashes and mood symptoms.

4. **Yasmin** contains 30 mcg of ethinyl estradiol and drospirenone. Drospirenone has anti-mineralocorticoid activity. It can help prevent bloating, weight gain, and hypertension, but it can increase serum potassium. Yasmin is contraindicated in patients at risk for hyperkalemia due to renal, hepatic, or adrenal disease. Yasmin should not be combined with other drugs that can increase potassium, such as ACE inhibitors, angiotensin receptor blockers, potassium-sparing diuretics, potassium supplements, NSAIDs, or salt substitutes.

5. **Third-generation progestins**
   a. More selective progestins include norgestimate, desogestrel, and gestodene. They have some structural modifications that lower their androgen activity. Norgestimate (eg, Ortho-Cyclen or Tri-Cyclen) and desogestrel (eg, Desogen or Ortho-Cept) are the least androgenic compounds in this class. The new progestins are not much less androgenic than norethindrone.
   b. The newer OCs are more effective in reducing acne and hirsutism in hyperandrogenic women. They are therefore an option for women who have difficulty tolerating older OCs. There is an increased risk of deep venous thrombosis with the use of these agents, and they should not be routinely used.

H. **Recommendations**
   1. Monophasic OCs containing the second generation progestin, norethindrone (Ovcon 35, Ortho-Novum 1/35) are recommended when starting a patient on OCs for the first time. This progestin has very low androgenicity when compared to other second generation progestins, and also compares favorably to the third generation progestins in androgenicity.
   2. The pill should be started on the first day of the period to provide the maximum contraceptive effect in the first cycle. However, most women start their pill on the first Sunday after the period starts. Some form of back-up contraception is needed for the first month if one chooses the Sunday start, because the full contraceptive effect might not be provided in the first pill pack.

Factors to Consider in Starting or Switching Oral Contraceptive Pills		
Objective	**Action**	**Products that achieve the objective**
To minimize high risk of thrombosis	Select a product with a lower dosage of estrogen.	Alesse, Aviane, Loestrin 1/20, Levlite, Mircette
To minimize nausea, breast tenderness or vascular headaches	Select a product with a lower dosage of estrogen.	Alesse, Aviane, Levlite, Loestrin 1/20, Mircette
To minimize spotting or breakthrough bleeding	Select a product with a higher dosage of estrogen or a progestin with greater potency.	Lo/Ovral, Nordette, Ortho-Cept, Ortho-Cyclen, Ortho Tri-Cyclen

Objective	Action	Products that achieve the objective
To minimize androgenic effects	Select a product containing a low-dose norethindrone or ethynodiol diacetate.	Brevicon, Demulen 1/35, Modicon, Ovcon 35
To avoid dyslipidemia	Select a product containing a low-dose norethindrone or ethynodiol diacetate.	Brevicon, Demulen 1/35, Modicon, Ovcon 35

Instructions on the Use of Oral Contraceptive Pills

Initiation of use (choose one):
The patient begins taking the pills on the first day of menstrual bleeding.
The patient begins taking the pills on the first Sunday after menstrual bleeding begins.
The patient begins taking the pills immediately if she is definitely not pregnant and has not had unprotected sex since her last menstrual period.

Missed pill
If it has been less than 24 hours since the last pill was taken, the patient takes a pill right away and then returns to normal pill-taking routine.
If it has been 24 hours since the last pill was taken, the patient takes both the missed pill and the next scheduled pill at the same time.
If it has been more than 24 hours since the last pill was taken (ie, two or more missed pills), the patient takes the last pill that was missed, throws out the other missed pills and takes the next pill on time. Additional contraception is used for the remainder of the cycle.

Additional contraceptive method
Use an additional contraceptive method for the first 7 days after initially starting oral contraceptive pills.
Use an additional contraceptive method for 7 days if more than 12 hours late in taking an oral contraceptive pill.
Use an additional contraceptive method while taking an interacting drug and for 7 days thereafter.

III. Injectable contraceptives

A. **Depot medroxyprogesterone acetate** (DMPA, Depo-Provera) is an injectable contraceptive. Deep intramuscular injection of 150 mg results in effective contraception for three to four months. Effectiveness is 99.7 percent.

B. Women who receive the first injection after the seventh day of the menstrual cycle should use a second method of contraception for seven days. The first injection should be administered within five days after the onset of menses, in which case alternative contraception is not necessary.

C. Ovulation is suppressed for at least 14 weeks after injection of a 150 mg dose of DMPA. Therefore, injections should repeated every three months. A pregnancy test must be administered to women who are more than two weeks late for an injection.

D. Return of fertility can be delayed for up to 18 months after cessation of DMPA. DMPA is not ideal for women who may wish to become pregnant soon after cessation of contraception.

E. Amenorrhea, irregular bleeding, and weight gain (typically 1 to 3 kg) are the most common adverse effects of DMPA. Adverse effects also include acne, headache, and depression. Fifty percent of women report amenorrhea by one year. Persistent bleeding may be treated with 50 µg of ethinyl estradiol for 14 days.

F. **Medroxyprogesterone acetate/estradiol cypionate (MPA/E2C, Lunelle)** is a combined (25 mg MPA and 5 mg E2C), injectable contraceptive.

1. Although monthly IM injections are required, MPA/E2C has several desirable features:
   a. It has nearly 100 percent effectiveness in preventing pregnancy.
   b. Fertility returns within three to four months after it is discontinued.
   c. Irregular bleeding is less common than in women given MPA alone.
2. Weight gain, hypertension, headache, mastalgia, or other nonmenstrual complaints are common.
3. Lunelle should be considered for women who forget to take their birth control pills or those who want a discreet method of contraception. The initial injection should be given during the first 5 days of the menstrual cycle or within 7 days of stopping oral contraceptives. Lunelle injections should be given every 28 to 30 days; 33 days at the most.

G. Transdermal contraceptive patch

1. **Ortho Evra** is a transdermal contraceptive patch, which is as effective as oral contraceptives. Ortho Evra delivers 20 μg of ethinyl estradiol and 150 μg of norelgestromin daily for 6 to 13 months. Compliance is better with the patch. The patch is applied at the beginning of the menstrual cycle. A new patch is applied each week for 3 weeks; week 4 is patch-free. It is sold in packages of 3 patches. Effectiveness is similar to oral contraceptives.
2. Breakthrough bleeding during the first two cycles, dysmenorrhea, and breast discomfort are more common in women using the patch. A reaction at the site of application of the patch occurs in 1.9 percent of the women. Contraceptive efficacy may be slightly lower in women weighing more than 90 kg.

H. Contraceptive vaginal ring (NuvaRing) delivers 15 μg ethinyl estradiol and 120 μg of etonogestrel daily. It is worn intravaginally for three weeks of each four week cycle. Advantages of this method include avoidance of gastrointestinal metabolism, rapid return to ovulation after discontinuation, lower doses of hormones, ease and convenience, and improved cycle control.

IV. Barrier methods

A. Barrier methods of contraception, such as the condom, diaphragm, cervical cap, and spermicides, have fewer side effects than hormonal contraception.
B. The diaphragm and cervical cap require fitting by a clinician and are only effective when used with a spermicide. They must be left in the vagina for six to eight hours after intercourse; the diaphragm needs to be removed after this period of time, while the cervical cap can be left in place for up to 24 hours. These considerations have caused them to be less desirable methods of contraception. A major advantage of barrier contraceptives is their efficacy in protecting against sexually transmitted diseases and HIV infection.

V. Intrauterine devices

A. The currently available intrauterine devices (IUDs) are safe and effective methods of contraception:
   1. **Copper T380 IUD** induces a foreign body reaction in the endometrium. It is effective for 8 to 10 years.
   2. **Progesterone-releasing IUDs** inhibit sperm survival and implantation. They also decrease menstrual blood loss and relieve dysmenorrhea. **Paragard** is replaced every 10 years. **Progestasert** IUDs must be replaced after one year.
   3. **Levonorgestrel IUD (Mirena)** provides effective contraception for five years.
B. Infection
   1. Women who are at low risk for sexually transmitted diseases do not have a higher incidence of pelvic inflammatory disease with use of an IUD. An IUD should not be inserted in women at high risk for sexually transmitted infections, and women should be screened for the presence of sexually transmitted diseases before insertion.
   2. **Contraindications to IUDs:**
      a. Women at high risk for bacterial endocarditis (eg, rheumatic heart

disease, prosthetic valves, or a history of endocarditis).
- **b.** Women at high risk for infections, including those with AIDS and a history of intravenous drug use.
- **c.** Women with uterine leiomyomas which alter the size or shape of the uterine cavity.

VI. Lactation
- **A.** Women who breast-feed have a delay in resumption of ovulation postpartum. It is probably safest to resume contraceptive use in the third postpartum month for those who breast-feed full time, and in the third postpartum week for those who do not breast-feed.
- **B.** A nonhormonal contraceptive or progesterone-containing hormonal contraceptive can be started at any time; an estrogen-containing oral contraceptive pill should not be started before the third week postpartum because women are still at increased risk of thromboembolism prior to this time. Oral contraceptive pills can decrease breast milk, while progesterone-containing contraceptives may increase breast milk.

VII. Progestin-only agents
- **A.** Progestin-only agents are slightly less effective than combination oral contraceptives. They have failure rates of 0.5 percent compared with the 0.1 percent rate with combination oral contraceptives.
- **B.** Progestin-only oral contraceptives (Micronor, Nor-QD, Ovrette) provide a useful alternative in women who cannot take estrogen. Progestin-only contraception is recommended for nursing mothers. Milk production is unaffected by use of progestin-only agents.
- **C.** If the usual time of ingestion is delayed for more than three hours, an alternative form of birth control should be used for the following 48 hours. Because progestin-only agents are taken continuously, without hormone-free periods, menses may be irregular, infrequent or absent.

VIII. Postcoital contraception
- **A.** Emergency postcoital contraception consists of administration of drugs within 72 hours to women who have had unprotected intercourse (including sexual assault), or to those who have had a failure of another method of contraception (eg, broken condom).
- **B.** Preparations
  1. Menstrual bleeding typically occurs within three days after administration of most forms of hormonal postcoital contraception. A pregnancy test should be performed if bleeding has not occurred within four weeks.
  2. **Preven Emergency Contraceptive Kit** includes four combination tablets, each containing 50 μg of ethinyl estradiol and 0.25 mg of levonorgestrel, and a pregnancy test to rule out pregnancy before taking the tablets. Instructions are to take two of the tablets as soon as possible within 72 hours of coitus, and the other two tablets twelve hours later.
  3. An oral contraceptive such as Ovral (two tablets twelve hours apart) or Lo/Ovral (4 tablets twelve hours apart) can also be used.
  4. Nausea and vomiting are the major side effects. Meclizine 50 mg, taken one hour before the first dose, reduces nausea and vomiting but can cause some sedation.
  5. **Plan B** is a pill pack that contains two 0.75 mg tablets of levonorgestrel to be taken twelve hours apart. The cost is comparable to the Preven kit ($20). This regimen may be more effective and better tolerated than an estrogen-progestin regimen.
  6. **Copper T380 IUD.** A copper intrauterine device (IUD) placed within 120 hours of unprotected intercourse can also be used as a form of emergency contraception. An advantage of this method is that it provides continuing contraception after the initial event.

Emergency Contraception

1. Consider pretreatment one hour before each oral contraceptive pill dose, using one of the following orally administered antiemetic agents:
   Prochlorperazine (Compazine), 5 to 10 mg
   Promethazine (Phenergan), 12.5 to 25 mg
   Trimethobenzamide (Tigan), 250 mg
   Meclizine (Antivert) 50 mg
2. Administer the first dose of oral contraceptive pill within 72 hours of unprotected coitus, and administer the second dose 12 hours after the first dose. Brand name options for emergency contraception include the following:
   Preven Kit – two pills per dose (0.5 mg of levonorgestrel and 100 µg of ethinyl estradiol per dose)
   Plan B – one pill per dose (0.75 mg of levonorgestrel per dose)
   Ovral – two pills per dose (0.5 mg of levonorgestrel and 100 µg of ethinyl estradiol per dose)
   Nordette – four pills per dose (0.6 mg of levonorgestrel and 120 µg of ethinyl estradiol per dose)
   Triphasil – four pills per dose (0.5 mg of levonorgestrel and 120 µg of ethinyl estradiol per dose)

References: See page 166.

Pregnancy Termination

Ninety percent of abortions are performed in the first trimester of pregnancy. About 1.5 million legal abortions are performed each year in the United States. Before 16 weeks of gestation, legal abortion may be performed in an office setting. Major anomalies and mid-trimester premature rupture of membranes are recognized fetal indications for termination.

I. Menstrual extraction
A. Many women seek abortion services within 1-2 weeks of the missed period. Abortion of these early pregnancies with a small-bore vacuum cannula is called menstrual extraction or minisuction. The only instruments required are a speculum, a tenaculum, a Karman cannula, and a modified 50 mL syringe.
B. The extracted tissue is rinsed and examined in a clear dish of water or saline over a light source to detect chorionic villi and the gestational sac. This examination is performed to rule out ectopic pregnancy and to decrease the risk of incomplete abortion.

II. First-trimester vacuum curettage
A. Beyond 7 menstrual weeks of gestation, larger cannulas and vacuum sources are required to evacuate a pregnancy. Vacuum curettage is the most common method of abortion. Procedures performed before 13 menstrual weeks are called suction or vacuum curettage, whereas similar procedures carried out after 13 weeks are termed dilation and evacuation.
B. Technique
   1. Uterine size and position should be assessed during a pelvic examination before the procedure. Ultrasonography is advised if there is a discrepancy of more than 2 weeks between the uterine size and menstrual dating.
   2. Tests for gonorrhea and chlamydia should be obtained, and the cervix and vagina should be prepared with a germicide. Paracervical block is established with 20 mL of 1% lidocaine injected deep into the cervix at the 3, 5, 7, and 9 o'clock positions. The cervix should be grasped with a single-toothed tenaculum placed vertically with one branch inside the canal. Uterine depth is measured with a sound. Dilation then should be performed with a tapered dilator.

3. A vacuum cannula with a diameter in millimeters that is one less than the estimated gestational age should be used to evacuate the cavity. After the tissue is removed, there should be a quick check with a sharp curette, followed by a brief reintroduction of the vacuum cannula. The aspirated tissue should be examined as described previously.

4. Antibiotics are used prophylactically. Doxycycline is the best agent because of a broad spectrum of antimicrobial effect. D-negative patients should receive D (Rho[D]) immune globulin.

C. Complications

1. The most common postabortal complications are pain, bleeding, and low-grade fever. Most cases are caused by retained gestational tissue or a clot in the uterine cavity. These symptoms are best managed by a repeat uterine evacuation, performed under local anesthesia

2. **Cervical shock.** Vasovagal syncope produced by stimulation of the cervical canal can be seen after paracervical block. Brief tonic-clonic activity rarely may be observed and is often confused with seizure. The routine use of atropine with paracervical anesthesia or the use of conscious sedation prevents cervical shock.

3. **Perforation**

   a. The risk of perforation is less than 1 in every 1,000 first-trimester abortions. It increases with gestational age and is greater for parous women than for nulliparous women. Perforation is best evaluated by laparoscopy to determine the extent of the injury.

   b. Perforations at the junction of the cervix and lower uterine segment can lacerate the ascending branch of the uterine artery within the broad ligament, giving rise to severe pain, a broad ligament hematoma, and intraabdominal bleeding. Management requires laparotomy, ligation of the severed vessels, and repair of the uterine injury.

4. **Hemorrhage**

   a. Excessive bleeding may indicate uterine atony, a low-lying implantation, a pregnancy of more advanced gestational age than the first trimester, or perforation. Management requires rapid reassessment of gestational age by examination of the fetal parts already extracted and gentle exploration of the uterine cavity with a curette and forceps. Intravenous oxytocin should be administered, and the abortion should be completed. The uterus then should be massaged to ensure contraction.

   b. When these measures fail, the patient should be hospitalized and should receive intravenous fluids and have her blood cross-matched. Persistent postabortal bleeding strongly suggests retained tissue or clot (hematometra) or trauma, and laparoscopy and repeat vacuum curettage is indicated.

5. **Hematometra.** Lower abdominal pain of increasing intensity in the first 30 minutes suggests hematometra. If there is no fever or bleeding is brisk, and on examination the uterus is large, globular, and tense, hematometra is likely. The treatment is immediate reevacuation.

6. **Ectopic pregnancy incomplete abortion, and failed abortion**

   a. Early detection of ectopic pregnancy, incomplete abortion, or failed abortion is possible with examination of the specimen immediately after the abortion. The patient may have an ectopic pregnancy if no chorionic villi are found. To detect an incomplete abortion that might result in continued pregnancy, the actual gestational sac must be identified.

   b. Determination of the b-hCG level and frozen section of the aspirated tissue and vaginal ultrasonography may be useful. If the b-hCG level is greater than 1,500-2,000 mIU, chorionic villi are not identified on frozen section, or retained tissue is identified by ultrasonography, immediate laparoscopy should be considered. Other patients may be followed closely with serial b-hCG assays until the problem is resolved. With later (>13 weeks) gestations, all of the fetal parts must be identified by the surgeon to prevent incomplete abortion.

c. Heavy bleeding or fever after abortion suggests retained tissue. If the postabortal uterus is larger than 12-week size, preoperative ultrasonography should be performed to determine the amount of remaining tissue. When fever is present, high-dose intravenous antibiotic therapy with two or three agents should be initiated, and curettage should be performed shortly thereafter.

III. **Mifepristone (RU-486) for medical abortion in the first trimester**

A. The FDA has approved mifepristone for termination of early pregnancy as follows: Eligible women are those whose last menstrual period began within the last 49 days. The patient takes 600 mg of mifepristone (three 200 mg tablets) by mouth on day 1, then 400 µg misoprostol orally two days later.

B. A follow-up visit is scheduled on day 14 to confirm that the pregnancy has been terminated with measurement of b-hCG or ultrasonography.

IV. **Second-trimester abortion.** Most abortions are performed before 13 menstrual weeks. Later abortions are generally performed because of fetal defects, maternal illness, or maternal age.

A. **Dilation and evacuation**

1. Transcervical dilation and evacuation of the uterus (D&E) is the method most commonly used for mid-trimester abortions before 21 menstrual weeks. In the one-stage technique, forcible dilation is performed slowly and carefully to sufficient diameter to allow insertion of large, strong ovum forceps for evacuation. The better approach is a two-stage procedure in which multiple Laminaria are used to achieve gradual dilatation over several hours before extraction. Uterine evacuation is accomplished with long, heavy forceps, using the vacuum cannula to rupture the fetal membranes, drain amniotic fluid, and ensure complete evacuation.

2. Preoperative ultrasonography is necessary for all cases 14 weeks and beyond. Intraoperative real-time ultrasonography helps to locate fetal parts within the uterus.

3. Dilation and evacuation becomes progressively more difficult as gestational age advances, and instillation techniques are often used after 21 weeks. Dilation and evacuation can be offered in the late mid-trimester, but two sets of Laminaria tents for a total of 36-48 hours is recommended. After multistage Laminaria treatment, urea is injected into the amniotic sac. Extraction is then accomplished after labor begins and after fetal maceration has occurred.

References: See page 166.

Ectopic Pregnancy

Ectopic pregnancy causes 15% of all maternal deaths. Once a patient has had an ectopic pregnancy, there is a 7- to 13-fold increase in the risk of recurrence.

I. **Clinical manifestations**

A. Symptoms of ectopic pregnancy include abdominal pain, amenorrhea, and vaginal bleeding. However, over 50 percent of women are asymptomatic before tubal rupture.

B. Symptoms of pregnancy (eg, breast tenderness, frequent urination, nausea) are often present. In cases of rupture, lightheadedness or shock may occur. EP should be suspected in any women of reproductive age with abdominal pain, especially those who have risk factors for an extrauterine pregnancy.

Risk Factors for Ectopic Pregnancy

Greatest Risk
Previous ectopic pregnancy
Previous tubal surgery or sterilization
Diethylstilbestrol exposure in utero
Documented tubal pathology (scarring)
Use of intrauterine contraceptive device

Greater Risk
Previous genital infections (eg, PID)
Infertility (In vitro fertilization)
Multiple sexual partners

Lesser Risk
Previous pelvic or abdominal surgery
Cigarette smoking
Vaginal douching
Age of 1st intercourse <18 years

Presenting Signs and Symptoms of Ectopic Pregnancy

Symptom	Percentage
Abdominal pain	80-100%
Amenorrhea	75-95%
Vaginal bleeding	50-80%
Dizziness, fainting	20-35%
Urge to defecate	5-15%
Pregnancy symptoms	10-25%
Passage of tissue	5-10%
Adnexal tenderness	75-90%
Abdominal tenderness	80-95%
Adnexal mass	50%
Uterine enlargement	20-30%
Orthostatic changes	10-15%
Fever	5-10%

C. **Physical examination.** Vital signs may reveal orthostatic changes and, occasionally, fever. Findings include adnexal and/or abdominal tenderness, an adnexal mass, and uterine enlargement.

II. **Diagnostic evaluation**
   A. Women with moderate- or high-risk factors for EP and those who conceived after in-vitro fertilization (IVF) should be evaluated for EP as soon as their first missed menses.
   B. **Transvaginal ultrasound** is most useful for identifying an intrauterine gestation. An extrauterine pregnancy will be visualized in only 16 to 32 percent of cases, thus a pelvic ultrasound showing "no intrauterine or extrauterine gestation" does not exclude the diagnosis of EP.
      1. The identification of an intrauterine pregnancy effectively excludes the possibility of an ectopic in almost all cases. However, pregnancies conceived with assisted reproductive technology are an exception, since the incidence of combined intrauterine and extrauterine pregnancy may be as high as 1/100 pregnancies.

2. An early intrauterine pregnancy is identified sonographically by the presence of a true gestational sac. Using TVS, the gestational sac is usually visible at 4.5 to 5 weeks of gestation with the double decidual sign at 5.5 to 6 weeks, the yolk sac appears at 5 to 6 weeks and remains until 10 weeks, and a fetal pole with cardiac activity is first detected at 5.5 to 6 weeks.

C. **beta-hCG concentration.** The gestational sac is usually identified at beta-hCG concentrations above 1500 to 2000 IU/L. The absence of an intrauterine gestational sac at beta-hCG concentrations above 2000 IU/L strongly suggests an EP.

D. **Progesterone** concentrations are higher in intrauterine than ectopic pregnancies. A concentration of greater than 25 ng/mL is usually (98 to 99 percent) associated with a viable intrauterine pregnancy, with lower concentrations in ectopic and intrauterine pregnancies that are destined to abort. A concentration less than 5 ng/mL almost always (99.8 percent) means the pregnancy is nonviable. However, there is no difference in the progesterone concentration between ectopic and arrested pregnancies. Progesterone measurements are useful only to confirm diagnostic impressions already obtained by hCG measurements and transvaginal sonography.

III. **Clinical decision making**

A. **Beta-hCG concentration greater than 1500 IU/L.** The interpretation of a beta-hCG at this level depends upon the findings on TVS.

   1. **Positive ultrasound.** Presence of an intrauterine pregnancy almost always excludes the presence of an EP. Fetal cardiac activity or a gestational sac with a clear fetal pole or yolk sac in an extrauterine location is diagnostic of an EP; treatment of EP should be initiated.

   2. **Negative ultrasound**
      a. An EP is very likely in the absence of an intrauterine pregnancy on TVS when the serum beta-hCG concentration is greater than 1500 IU/L. The next step is to confirm the diagnostic impression by repeating the TVS examination and beta-hCG concentration two days later. The diagnosis of EP is certain at this time if an intrauterine pregnancy is not observed on TVS and the serum beta-hCG concentration is increasing or plateaued. Treatment of EP should be initiated.
      b. A falling beta-hCG concentration is most consistent with a failed pregnancy (eg, arrested pregnancy, blighted ovum, tubal abortion, spontaneously resolving EP). Weekly beta-hCG concentrations should be monitored until the result is negative for pregnancy.

B. **Beta-hCG concentration greater than 1500 IU/L and an adnexal mass.** An extrauterine pregnancy is almost certain when the serum beta-hCG concentration is greater than 1500 IU/L, a nonspecific adnexal mass is present, and no intrauterine pregnancy is observed on TVS. Treatment of EP should be initiated.

C. **Beta-hCG less than 1500 IU/L**

   1. A serum beta-hCG concentration less than 1500 IU/L with a TVS examination that is negative should be followed by repetition of both of these tests in three days to follow the rate of rise of the hCG. Beta-hCG concentrations usually double every 1.5 to two days until six to seven weeks of gestation in viable intrauterine pregnancies (and in some ectopic gestations). A beta-hCG concentration that does not double over 72 hours associated with a repeat TVS examination that does not show an intrauterine gestation means that the pregnancy is nonviable, such as an ectopic gestation or intrauterine pregnancy that is destined to abort. A normal intrauterine pregnancy is not present and medical treatment of EP can be initiated.

   2. A normally rising beta-hCG concentration should be evaluated with TVS until an intrauterine pregnancy or an ectopic pregnancy can be demonstrated.

   3. A falling beta-hCG concentration is most consistent with a failed pregnancy (eg, arrested pregnancy, blighted ovum, tubal abortion,

spontaneously resolving EP). Weekly beta-hCG concentrations should be monitored until the result is negative for pregnancy.

IV. **Methotrexate therapy for ectopic pregnancy**
  A. Medical treatment of ectopic pregnancy (EP) with methotrexate (MTX) has supplanted surgical therapy in most cases. The success rate is 86 to 94 percent.
  B. Methotrexate is a folic acid antagonist, which inhibits DNA synthesis and cell reproduction.

Criteria for Receiving Methotrexate

Absolute indications
Hemodynamically stable without active bleeding or signs of hemoperitoneum
Nonlaparoscopic diagnosis
Patient desires future fertility
General anesthesia poses a significant risk
Patient is able to return for follow-up care
Patient has no contraindications to methotrexate

Relative indications
Unruptured mass <3.5 cm at its greatest dimension
No fetal cardiac motion detected
Patients whose bet-hCG level does not exceed 6,000-15,000 mIU/mL

Contraindications to Methotrexate Therapy

Absolute contraindications
Breast feeding
Overt or laboratory evidence of immunodeficiency
Alcoholism, alcoholic liver disease, or other chronic liver disease
Preexisting blood dyscrasias, such as bone marrow hypoplasia, leukopenia, thrombocytopenia, or significant anemia
Known sensitivity to methotrexate
Active pulmonary disease
Peptic ulcer disease
Hepatic, renal, or hematologic dysfunction
Relative contraindications
Gestational sac >3.5 cm
Embryonic cardiac motion

  C. **Contraindications to medical treatment**
    1. Women who are hemodynamically unstable, not likely to be compliant with post-therapeutic monitoring, and who do not have timely access to a medical institution should be treated surgically.
    2. The presence of fetal cardiac activity is a relative contraindication to medical treatment.
    3. Women with a high baseline hCG concentration (>5000 mIU/mL) are more likely to experience treatment failure; they may be better served by conservative laparoscopic surgery.
  D. **Protocol**
    1. **Single dose therapy.** A single intramuscular dose of methotrexate (50 mg per square meter of body surface area) is given. The body surface area (BSA) may be calculated based upon height and weight.
    2. **RhoGAM** should be administered if the woman is Rh(D)-negative and the blood group of her male partner is Rh(D)-positive or unknown.
  E. **Adverse reactions** to MTX are usually mild and self-limiting. The most common are stomatitis and conjunctivitis. Rare side effects include gastritis, enteritis, dermatitis, pleuritis, alopecia, elevated liver enzymes, and bone marrow suppression.
  F. **Post-therapy monitoring and evaluation**. Serum beta-hCG concentration and ultrasound examination should be evaluated weekly. An increase in beta-hCG levels in the three days following therapy (ie, up to day 4)

and mild abdominal pain of short duration (one to two days) are common. The pain can be controlled with nonsteroidal antiinflammatory drugs.

G. A second dose of methotrexate should be administered if the serum beta-hCG concentration on Day 7 has not declined by at least 25 percent from the Day 0 level. Approximately 20 percent of women will require a second dose of MTX.

H. The beta-hCG concentration usually declines to less than 15 mIU/mL by 35 days post-injection, but may take as long as 109 days. Weekly assays should be obtained until this level is reached.

Side Effects Associated with Methotrexate Treatment	
Increase in abdominal pain (occurs in up to two-thirds of patients)	Gastric distress
Nausea	Dizziness
Vomiting	Vaginal bleeding or spotting
Stomatitis	Severe neutropenia (rare)
Diarrhea	Reversible alopecia (rare)
	Pneumonitis

Signs of Treatment Failure and Tubal Rupture
Significantly worsening abdominal pain, regardless of change in beta-hCG levels
Hemodynamic instability
Levels of beta-hCG that do not decline by at least 15% between day 4 and day 7 postinjection
Increasing or plateauing beta-hCG levels after the first week of treatment

V. Operative management can be accomplished by either laparoscopy or laparotomy. Linear salpingostomy or segmental resection is the procedure of choice if the fallopian tube is to be retained. Salpingectomy is the procedure of choice if the tube requires removal.

References: See page 166.

Acute Pelvic Pain

I. Clinical evaluation

  A. Assessment of acute pelvic pain should determine the patient's age, obstetrical history, menstrual history, characteristics of pain onset, duration, and palliative or aggravating factors.

  B. Associated symptoms may include urinary or gastrointestinal symptoms, fever, abnormal bleeding, or vaginal discharge.

  C. Past medical history. Contraceptive history, surgical history, gynecologic history, history of pelvic inflammatory disease, ectopic pregnancy, sexually transmitted diseases should be determined. Current sexual activity and practices should be assessed.

  D. Method of contraception

    1. Sexual abstinence in the months preceding the onset of pain lessons the likelihood of pregnancy-related etiologies.

    2. The risk of acute PID is reduced by 50% in patients taking oral contraceptives or using a barrier method of contraception. Patients taking oral contraceptives are at decreased risk for an ectopic pregnancy or ovarian cysts.

  E. Risk factors for acute pelvic inflammatory disease. Age between 15-25 years, sexual partner with symptoms of urethritis, prior history of PID.

II. Physical examination

  A. Fever, abdominal or pelvic tenderness, and peritoneal signs should be sought.

B. Vaginal discharge, cervical erythema and discharge, cervical and uterine motion tenderness, or adnexal masses or tenderness should be noted.

III. **Laboratory tests**

A. **Pregnancy testing** will identify pregnancy-related causes of pelvic pain. Serum beta-HCG becomes positive 7 days after conception. A negative test virtually excludes ectopic pregnancy.

B. **Complete blood count.** Leukocytosis suggest an inflammatory process; however, a normal white blood count occurs in 56% of patients with PID and 37% of patients with appendicitis.

C. **Urinalysis.** The finding of pyuria suggests urinary tract infection. Pyuria can also occur with an inflamed appendix or from contamination of the urine by vaginal discharge.

D. **Testing for Neisseria gonorrhoeae and Chlamydia trachomatis** are necessary if PID is a possibility.

E. **Pelvic ultrasonography** is of value in excluding the diagnosis of an ectopic pregnancy by demonstrating an intrauterine gestation. Sonography may reveal acute PID, torsion of the adnexa, or acute appendicitis.

F. **Diagnostic laparoscopy** is indicated when acute pelvic pain has an unclear diagnosis despite comprehensive evaluation.

III. **Differential diagnosis of acute pelvic pain**

A. **Pregnancy-related causes.** Ectopic pregnancy, spontaneous, threatened or incomplete abortion, intrauterine pregnancy with corpus luteum bleeding.

B. **Gynecologic disorders.** PID, endometriosis, ovarian cyst hemorrhage or rupture, adnexal torsion, Mittelschmerz, uterine leiomyoma torsion, primary dysmenorrhea, tumor.

C. **Nonreproductive tract causes**

1. **Gastrointestinal.** Appendicitis, inflammatory bowel disease, mesenteric adenitis, irritable bowel syndrome, diverticulitis.

2. **Urinary tract.** Urinary tract infection, renal calculus.

IV. **Approach to acute pelvic pain with a positive pregnancy test**

A. In a female patient of reproductive age, presenting with acute pelvic pain, the first distinction is whether the pain is pregnancy-related or non-pregnancy-related on the basis of a serum pregnancy test.

B. In the patient with acute pelvic pain associated with pregnancy, the next step is localization of the tissue responsible for the hCG production. Transvaginal ultrasound should be performed to identify an intrauterine gestation. Ectopic pregnancy is characterized by a noncystic adnexal mass and fluid in the cul-de-sac.

V. **Approach to acute pelvic pain in non-pregnant patients with a negative HCG**

A. **Acute PID** is the leading diagnostic consideration in patients with acute pelvic pain unrelated to pregnancy. The pain is usually bilateral, but may be unilateral in 10%. Cervical motion tenderness, fever, and cervical discharge are common findings.

B. **Acute appendicitis** should be considered in all patients presenting with acute pelvic pain and a negative pregnancy test. Appendicitis is characterized by leukocytosis and a history of a few hours of periumbilical pain followed by migration of the pain to the right lower quadrant. Neutrophilia occurs in 75%. A slight fever exceeding 37.3°C, nausea, vomiting, anorexia, and rebound tenderness may be present.

C. **Torsion of the adnexa** usually causes unilateral pain, but pain can be bilateral in 25%. Intense, progressive pain combined with a tense, tender adnexal mass is characteristic. There is often a history of repetitive, transitory pain. Pelvic sonography often confirms the diagnosis. Laparoscopic diagnosis and surgical intervention are indicated.

D. **Ruptured or hemorrhagic corpus luteal cyst** usually causes bilateral pain, but it can cause unilateral tenderness in 35%. Ultrasound aids in diagnosis.

E. **Endometriosis** usually causes chronic or recurrent pain, but it can occasionally cause acute pelvic pain. There usually is a history of dysmenorrhea and deep dyspareunia. Pelvic exam reveals fixed uterine retrodisplacement and tender uterosacral and cul-de-sac nodularity. Laparoscopy confirms the diagnosis.

References: See page 166.

Chronic Pelvic Pain

Chronic pelvic pain (CPP) affects approximately one in seven women in the United States (14 percent). Chronic pelvic pain (>6 months in duration) is less likely to be associated with a readily identifiable cause than is acute pain.

I. **Etiology of chronic pelvic pain**
   A. **Physical and sexual abuse.** Numerous studies have demonstrated a higher frequency of physical and/or sexual abuse in women with CPP. Between 30 and 50 percent of women with CPP have a history of abuse (physical or sexual, childhood or adult).
   B. **Gynecologic problems**
      1. **Endometriosis** is present in approximately one-third of women undergoing laparoscopy for CPP and is the most frequent finding in these women. Typically, endometriosis pain is a sharp or "crampy" pain. It starts at the onset of menses, becoming more severe and prolonged over several menstrual cycles. It is frequently accompanied by deep dyspareunia. Uterosacral ligament nodularity is highly specific for endometriosis. Examining the woman during her menstruation may make the nodularity easier to palpate. A more common, but less specific, finding is tenderness in the cul-de-sac or uterosacral ligaments that reproduces the pain of deep dyspareunia.
      2. **Pelvic adhesions** are found in approximately one-fourth of women undergoing laparoscopy for CPP. Adhesions form after intra-abdominal inflammation; they should be suspected if the woman has a history of surgery or pelvic inflammatory disease (PID). The pain may be a dull or sharp pulling sensation that occurs at any time during the month. Physical examination is usually nondiagnostic.
      3. **Dysmenorrhea** (painful menstruation) and mittelschmerz (midcycle pain) without other organic pathology are seen frequently and may contribute to CPP in more than half of all cases.
      4. **Chronic pelvic inflammatory disease** may cause CPP. Therefore, culturing for sexually transmitted agents should be a routine part of the evaluation.

Medical Diagnoses and Chronic Pelvic Pain	
Medical diagnosis/symptom source	**Prevalence**
Bowel dysmotility disorders	50 to 80%
Musculoskeletal disorders	30 to 70%
Cyclic gynecologic pain	20 to 50%
Urologic diagnoses	5 to 10%
Endometriosis, advanced and/or with dense bowel adhesions	Less than 5%
Unusual medical diagnoses	Less than 2%
Multiple medical diagnoses	30 to 50%
No identifiable medical diagnosis	Less than 5%

   C. **Nongynecologic medical problems**
      1. **Bowel dysmotility** (eg, irritable bowel syndrome and constipation) may be the primary symptom source in 50 percent of all cases of CPP and may be a contributing factor in up to 80 percent of cases. Pain from irritable bowel syndrome is typically described as a crampy, recurrent pain accompanied by abdominal distention and bloating,

alternating diarrhea and constipation, and passage of mucus. The pain is often worse during or near the menstrual period. A highly suggestive sign is exquisite tenderness to palpation which improves with continued pressure.

2. **Musculoskeletal dysfunction,** including abdominal myofascial pain syndromes, can cause or contribute to CPP.

D. **Psychologic problems**

1. **Depressive disorders** contribute to more than half of all cases of CPP. Frequently, the pain becomes part of a cycle of pain, disability, and mood disturbance. The diagnostic criteria for depression include depressed mood, diminished interest in daily activities, weight loss or gain, insomnia or hypersomnia, psychomotor agitation or retardation, fatigue, feelings of worthlessness, loss of concentration, and recurrent thoughts of death.

2. **Somatoform disorders,** including somatization disorder, contribute to 10 to 20 percent of cases of CPP. The essential feature of somatization disorder is a pattern of recurring, multiple, clinically significant somatic complaints.

II. **Clinical evaluation of chronic pelvic pain**

A. **History**

1. The character, intensity, distribution, and location of pain are important. Radiation of pain or should be assessed. The temporal pattern of the pain (onset, duration, changes, cyclicity) and aggravating or relieving factors (eg, posture, meals, bowel movements, voiding, menstruation, intercourse, medications) should be documented.

2. **Associated symptoms.** Anorexia, constipation, or fatigue are often present.

3. **Previous surgeries,** pelvic infections, infertility, or obstetric experiences may provide additional clues.

4. For patients of reproductive age, the timing and characteristics of their last menstrual period, the presence of non-menstrual vaginal bleeding or discharge, and the method of contraception used should be determined.

5. Life situations and events that affect the pain should be sought.

6. Gastrointestinal and urologic symptoms, including the relationship between these systems to the pain should be reviewed.

7. The patient's affect may suggest depression or other mood disorders.

B. **Physical examination**

1. If the woman indicates the location of her pain with a single finger, the pain is more likely caused by a discrete source than if she uses a sweeping motion of her hand.

2. A pelvic examination should be performed. Special attention should be given to the bladder, urethra.

3. The piriformis muscles should be palpated; piriformis spasm can cause pain when climbing stairs, driving a car, or when first arising in the morning. This muscle is responsible for external rotation of the hip and can be palpated posterolaterally, cephalic to the ischial spine. This examination is most easily performed if the woman externally rotates her hip against the resistance of the examiner's other hand. Piriformis spasm is treated with physical therapy.

4. Abdominal deformity, erythema, edema, scars, hernias, or distension should be noted. Abnormal bowel sounds may suggest a gastrointestinal process.

5. Palpation should include the epigastrium, flanks, and low back, and inguinal areas.

C. **Special tests**

1. Initial laboratory tests should include cervical cytology, endocervical cultures for *Neisseria gonorrhoeae* and Chlamydia, stool Hemoccult, and urinalysis. Other tests may be suggested by the history and examination.

2. Laparoscopy is helpful when the pelvic examination is abnormal or when initial therapy fails.

III. Management

A. Myofascial pain syndrome may be treated by a variety of physical therapy techniques. Trigger points can often be treated with injections of a local anesthetic (eg, bupivacaine [Marcaine]), with or without the addition of a corticosteroid.

B. If the pain is related to the menstrual cycle, treatment aimed at suppressing the cycle may help. Common methods to accomplish this include administration of depot medroxyprogesterone (Depo-Provera) and continuously dosed oral contraceptives.

C. Cognitive-behavioral therapy is appropriate for all women with CPP. Relaxation and distraction techniques are often helpful.

D. When endometriosis or pelvic adhesions are discovered on diagnostic laparoscopy, they are usually treated during the procedure. Hysterectomy may be warranted if the pain has persisted for more than six months, does not respond to analgesics (including anti-inflammatory agents), and impairs the woman's normal function.

E. Antidepressants or sleeping aids are useful adjunctive therapies. Amitriptyline (Elavil), in low doses of 25-50 mg qhs, may be of help in improving sleep and reducing the severity of chronic pain complaints.

F. Muscle relaxants may prove useful in patients with guarding, splinting, or reactive muscle spasms.

References: See page 166.

Endometriosis

Endometriosis is characterized by the presence of endometrial tissue on the ovaries, fallopian tubes or other abnormal sites, causing pain or infertility. Women are usually 25 to 29 years old at the time of diagnosis. Approximately 24 percent of women who complain of pelvic pain are subsequently found to have endometriosis. The overall prevalence of endometriosis is estimated to be 5 to 10 percent.

I. Clinical evaluation

A. Endometriosis should be considered in any woman of reproductive age who has pelvic pain. The most common symptoms are dysmenorrhea, dyspareunia, and low back pain that worsens during menses. Rectal pain and painful defecation may also occur. Other causes of secondary dysmenorrhea and chronic pelvic pain (eg, upper genital tract infections, adenomyosis, adhesions) may produce similar symptoms.

Differential Diagnosis of Endometriosis

Generalized pelvic pain
Pelvic inflammatory disease
Endometritis
Pelvic adhesions
Neoplasms, benign or malignant
Ovarian torsion
Sexual or physical abuse
Nongynecologic causes

Dysmenorrhea
Primary
Secondary (adenomyosis, myomas, infection, cervical stenosis)

Dyspareunia
Musculoskeletal causes (pelvic relaxation, levator spasm)
Gastrointestinal tract (constipation, irritable bowel syndrome)
Urinary tract (urethral syndrome, interstitial cystitis)
Infection
Pelvic vascular congestion
Diminished lubrication or vaginal expansion because of insufficient arousal

Infertility
Male factor
Tubal disease (infection)
Anovulation
Cervical factors (mucus, sperm antibodies, stenosis)
Luteal phase deficiency

B. Infertility may be the presenting complaint for endometriosis. Infertile patients often have no painful symptoms.

C. Physical examination. The physician should palpate for a fixed, retroverted uterus, adnexal and uterine tenderness, pelvic masses or nodularity along the uterosacral ligaments. A rectovaginal examination should identify uterosacral, cul-de-sac or septal nodules. Most women with endometriosis have normal pelvic findings.

II. Treatment

A. Confirmatory laparoscopy is usually required before treatment is instituted. In women with few symptoms, an empiric trial of oral contraceptives or progestins may be warranted to assess pain relief.

B. Medical treatment

1. Initial therapy also should include a nonsteroidal anti-inflammatory drug.
   a. Naproxen (Naprosyn) 500 mg followed by 250 mg PO tid-qid prn [250, 375,500 mg].
   b. Naproxen sodium (Aleve) 200 mg PO tid prn.
   c. Naproxen sodium (Anaprox) 550 mg, followed by 275 mg PO tid-qid prn.
   d. Ibuprofen (Motrin) 800 mg, then 400 mg PO q4-6h prn.
   e. Mefenamic acid (Ponstel) 500 mg PO followed by 250 mg q6h prn.

2. **Progestational agents.** Progestins are similar to combination OCPs in their effects on FSH, LH and endometrial tissue. They may be associated with more bothersome adverse effects than OCPs. Progestins are effective in reducing the symptoms of endometriosis. Oral progestin regimens may include once-daily administration of medroxyprogesterone at the lowest effective dosage (5 to 20 mg). Depot medroxyprogesterone may be given intramuscularly every two weeks for two months at 100 mg per dose and then once a month for four months at 200 mg per dose.

3. **Oral contraceptive pills (OCPs)** suppress LH and FSH and prevent ovulation. Combination OCPs alleviate symptoms in about three quarters of patients. Oral contraceptives can be taken continuously (with no placebos) or cyclically, with a week of placebo pills between cycles. The OCPs can be discontinued after six months or continued indefinitely.

4. **Danazol (Danocrine)** has been highly effective in relieving the symptoms of endometriosis, but adverse effects may preclude its use. Adverse effects include headache, flushing, sweating and atrophic vaginitis. Androgenic side effects include acne, edema, hirsutism, deepening of the voice and weight gain. The initial dosage should be 800 mg per day, given in two divided oral doses. The overall response rate is 84 to 92 percent.

Medical Treatment of Endometriosis		
Drug	**Dosage**	**Adverse effects**
Danazol (Danocrine)	800 mg per day in 2 divided doses	Estrogen deficiency, androgenic side effects
Oral contraceptives	1 pill per day (continuous or cyclic)	Headache, nausea, hypertension
Medroxyprogesterone (Provera)	5 to 20 mg orally per day	Same as with other oral progestins

Drug	Dosage	Adverse effects
Medroxyproges-terone suspension (Depo-Provera)	100 mg IM every 2 weeks for 2 months; then 200 mg IM every month for 4 months or 150 mg IM every 3 months	Weight gain, depression, irregular menses or amenorrhea
Norethindrone (Aygestin)	5 mg per day orally for 2 weeks; then increase by 2.5 mg per day every 2 weeks up to 15 mg per day	Same as with other oral progestins
Leuprolide (Lupron)	3.75 mg IM every month for 6 months	Decrease in bone density, estrogen deficiency
Goserelin (Zoladex)	3.6 mg SC (in upper abdominal wall) every 28 days	Estrogen deficiency
Nafarelin (Synarel)	400 mg per day: 1 spray in 1 nostril in a.m.; 1 spray in other nostril in p.m.; start treatment on day 2 to 4 of menstrual cycle	Estrogen deficiency, bone density changes, nasal irritation

    C. GnRH agonists. These agents (eg, leuprolide [Lupron], goserelin [Zoladex]) inhibit the secretion of gonadotropin. GnRH agonists are contraindicated in pregnancy and have hypoestrogenic side effects. They produce a mild degree of bone loss. Because of concerns about osteopenia, "add-back" therapy with low-dose estrogen has been recommended. The dosage of leuprolide is a single monthly 3.75-mg depot injection given intramuscularly. Goserelin, in a dosage of 3.6 mg, is administered subcutaneously every 28 days. A nasal spray (nafarelin [Synarel]) may be used twice daily. The response rate is similar to that with danazol; about 90 percent of patients experience pain relief.

    D. Surgical treatment
      1. Surgical treatment is the preferred approach to infertile patients with advanced endometriosis. Laparoscopic ablation of endometriosis lesions may result in a 13 percent increase in the probability of pregnancy.
      2. Definitive surgery, which includes hysterectomy and oophorectomy, is reserved for women with intractable pain who no longer desire pregnancy.

References: See page 166.

Primary Amenorrhea

Amenorrhea (absence of menses) results from dysfunction of the hypothalamus, pituitary, ovaries, uterus, or vagina. It is often classified as either primary (absence of menarche by age 16) or secondary (absence of menses for more than three cycle intervals or six months in women who were previously menstruating).

I. Etiology
    A. Primary amenorrhea is usually the result of a genetic or anatomic abnormality. Common etiologies of primary amenorrhea:
      1. Chromosomal abnormalities causing gonadal dysgenesis: 45 percent
      2. Physiologic delay of puberty: 20 percent
      3. Müllerian agenesis: 15 percent
      4. Transverse vaginal septum or imperforate hymen: 5 percent
      5. Absent production of gonadotropin-releasing hormone (GnRH) by the hypothalamus: 5 percent

6. Anorexia nervosa: 2 percent
7. Hypopituitarism: 2 percent

Causes of Primary and Secondary Amenorrhea

Abnormality	Causes
Pregnancy	
Anatomic abnormalities	
Congenital abnormality in Mullerian development	Isolated defect Testicular feminization syndrome 5-Alpha-reductase deficiency Vanishing testes syndrome Defect in testis determining factor
Congenital defect of urogenital sinus development	Agenesis of lower vagina Imperforate hymen
Acquired ablation or scarring of the endometrium	Asherman's syndrome Tuberculosis
Disorders of hypothalamic-pituitary ovarian axis Hypothalamic dysfunction Pituitary dysfunction Ovarian dysfunction	

Causes of Amenorrhea due to Abnormalities in the Hypothalamic-Pituitary-Ovarian Axis

Abnormality	Causes

Hypothalamic dysfunction	Functional hypothalamic amenorrhea
	    Weight loss, eating disorders
	    Exercise
	    Stress
	    Severe or prolonged illness
	Congenital gonadotropin-releasing hormone deficiency
	Inflammatory or infiltrative diseases
	Brain tumors - eg, craniopharyngioma
	Pituitary stalk dissection or compression
	Cranial irradiation
	Brain injury - trauma, hemorrhage, hydrocephalus
	Other syndromes - Prader-Willi, Laurence-Moon-Biedl

Pituitary dysfunction	Hyperprolactinemia Other pituitary tumors- acromegaly, corticotroph adenomas (Cushing's disease) Other tumors - meningioma, germinoma, glioma Empty sella syndrome Pituitary infarct or apoplexy

Ovarian dysfunction	Ovarian failure (menopause)
	    Spontaneous
	    Premature (before age 40 years)
	    Surgical

Abnormality	Causes
Other	Hyperthyroidism Hypothyroidism Diabetes mellitus Exogenous androgen use

II. Diagnostic evaluation of primary amenorrhea

A. Step I: Evaluate clinical history:

1. Signs of puberty may include a growth spurt, absence of axillary and pubic hair, or apocrine sweat glands, or absence of breast development. Lack of pubertal development suggests ovarian or pituitary failure or a chromosomal abnormality.
2. Family history of delayed or absent puberty suggests a familial disorder.
3. Short stature may indicate Turner syndrome or hypothalamic-pituitary disease.
4. Poor health may be a manifestation of hypothalamic-pituitary disease. Symptoms of other hypothalamic-pituitary disease include headaches, visual field defects, fatigue, or polyuria and polydipsia.
5. Virilization suggests polycystic ovary syndrome, an androgen-secreting ovarian or adrenal tumor, or the presence of Y chromosome material.
6. Recent stress, change in weight, diet, or exercise habits; or illness may suggest hypothalamic amenorrhea.
7. Heroin and methadone can alter hypothalamic gonadotropin secretion.
8. Galactorrhea is suggestive of excess prolactin. Some drugs cause amenorrhea by increasing serum prolactin concentrations, including metoclopramide and antipsychotic drugs.

B. Step II: Physical examination

1. An evaluation of pubertal development should include current height, weight, and arm span (normal arm span for adults is within 5 cm of height) and an evaluation of the growth chart.
2. Breast development should be assessed by Tanner staging.
3. The genital examination should evaluate clitoral size, pubertal hair development, intactness of the hymen, depth of the vagina, and presence of a cervix, uterus, and ovaries. If the vagina can not be penetrated with a finger, rectal examination may allow evaluation of the internal organs. Pelvic ultrasound is also useful to determine the presence or absence of müllerian structures.
4. The skin should be examined for hirsutism, acne, striae, increased pigmentation, and vitiligo.
5. Classic physical features of Turner syndrome include low hair line, web neck, shield chest, and widely spaced nipples.

C. Step III: Basic laboratory testing

1. **If a normal vagina or uterus are not obviously present** on physical examination, pelvic ultrasonography should be performed to confirm the presence or absence of ovaries, uterus, and cervix. Ultrasonography can be useful to exclude vaginal or cervical outlet obstruction in patients with cyclic pain.

   a. **Uterus absent**
      (1) If the uterus is absent, evaluation should include a karyotype and serum testosterone. These tests should distinguish abnormal müllerian development (46,XX karyotype with normal female serum testosterone concentrations) from androgen insensitivity syndrome (46,XY karyotype and normal male serum testosterone concentrations).
      (2) Patients with 5-alpha reductase deficiency also have a 46,XY karyotype and normal male serum testosterone concentrations

but, in contrast to the androgen insensitivity syndrome which is associated with a female phenotype, these patients undergo striking virilization at the time of puberty (secondary sexual hair, muscle mass, and deepening of the voice).

2. **Uterus present.** For patients with a normal vagina and uterus and no evidence of an imperforate hymen, vaginal septum, or congenital absence of the vagina. Measurement of serum beta human chorionic gonadotropin to exclude pregnancy and of serum FSH, prolactin, and TSH.

   a. A high serum FSH concentration is indicative of primary ovarian failure. A karyotype is then required and may demonstrate complete or partial deletion of the X chromosome (Turner syndrome) or the presence of Y chromatin. The presence of a Y chromosome is associated with a higher risk of gonadal tumors and makes gonadectomy mandatory.

   b. A low or normal serum FSH concentration suggests functional hypothalamic amenorrhea, congenital GnRH deficiency, or other disorders of the hypothalamic-pituitary axis. Cranial MR imaging is indicated in most cases of hypogonadotropic hypogonadism to evaluate hypothalamic or pituitary disease. Cranial MRI is recommended for all women with primary hypogonadotropic hypogonadism, visual field defects, or headaches.

   c. Serum prolactin and thyrotropin (TSH) should be measured, especially if galactorrhea is present.

   d. If there are signs or symptoms of hirsutism, serum testosterone and dehydroepiandrosterone sulfate (DHEA-S) should be measured to assess for an androgen-secreting tumor.

   e. If hypertension is present, blood tests should be drawn for evaluate for CYP17 deficiency. The characteristic findings are elevations in serum progesterone (>3 ng/mL) and deoxycorticosterone and low values for serum 17-alpha-hydroxyprogesterone (<0.2 ng/mL).

III. Treatment

A. Treatment of primary amenorrhea is directed at correcting the underlying pathology; helping the woman to achieve fertility, if desired; and prevention of complications of the disease.

B. **Congenital anatomic lesions or Y chromosome material** usually requires surgery. Surgical correction of a vaginal outlet obstruction is necessary before menarche, or as soon as the diagnosis is made after menarche. Creation of a neovagina for patients with müllerian failure is usually delayed until the women are emotionally mature. If Y chromosome material is found, gonadectomy should be performed to prevent gonadal neoplasia. However, gonadectomy should be delayed until after puberty in patients with androgen insensitivity syndrome. These patients have a normal pubertal growth spurt and feminize at the time of expected puberty.

C. **Ovarian failure** requires counseling about the benefits and risks of hormone replacement therapy.

D. **Polycystic ovary syndrome** is managed with measures to reduce hirsutism, resume menses, and fertility and prevent of endometrial hyperplasia, obesity, and metabolic defects.

E. **Functional hypothalamic amenorrhea** can usually be reversed by weight gain, reduction in the intensity of exercise, or resolution of illness or emotional stress. For women who want to continue to exercise, estrogen-progestin replacement therapy should be given to those not seeking fertility to prevent osteoporosis. Women who want to become pregnant can be treated with gonadotropins or pulsatile GnRH.

F. **Hypothalamic or pituitary dysfunction** that is not reversible (eg, congenital GnRH deficiency) is treated with either exogenous gonadotropins or pulsatile GnRH if the woman wants to become pregnant.

References: See page 166.

Secondary Amenorrhea

Amenorrhea (absence of menses) can be a transient, intermittent, or permanent condition resulting from dysfunction of the hypothalamus, pituitary, ovaries, uterus, or vagina. Amenorrhea is classified as either primary (absence of menarche by age 16 years) or secondary (absence of menses for more than three cycles or six months in women who previously had menses). Pregnancy is the most common cause of secondary amenorrhea.

I. Diagnosis

A. **Step 1: Rule out pregnancy**. A pregnancy test is the first step in evaluating secondary amenorrhea. Measurement of serum beta subunit of hCG is the most sensitive test.

B. **Step 2: Assess the history**

1. Recent stress; change in weight, diet or exercise habits; or illnesses that might result in hypothalamic amenorrhea should be sought.
2. Drugs associated with amenorrhea, systemic illnesses that can cause hypothalamic amenorrhea, recent initiation or discontinuation of an oral contraceptive, androgenic drugs (danazol) or high-dose progestin, and antipsychotic drugs should be evaluated.
3. Headaches, visual field defects, fatigue, or polyuria and polydipsia may suggest hypothalamic-pituitary disease.
4. Symptoms of estrogen deficiency include hot flashes, vaginal dryness, poor sleep, or decreased libido.
5. Galactorrhea is suggestive of hyperprolactinemia. Hirsutism, acne, and a history of irregular menses are suggestive of hyperandrogenism.
6. A history of obstetrical catastrophe, severe bleeding, dilatation and curettage, or endometritis or other infection that might have caused scarring of the endometrial lining suggests Asherman's syndrome.

Causes of Primary and Secondary Amenorrhea	
Abnormality	**Causes**
Pregnancy	
Anatomic abnormalities	
Congenital abnormality in Mullerian development	Isolated defect Testicular feminization syndrome 5-Alpha-reductase deficiency Vanishing testes syndrome Defect in testis determining factor
Congenital defect of urogenital sinus development	Agenesis of lower vagina Imperforate hymen
Acquired ablation or scarring of the endometrium	Asherman's syndrome Tuberculosis
Disorders of hypothalamic-pituitary ovarian axis Hypothalamic dysfunction Pituitary dysfunction Ovarian dysfunction	

Causes of Amenorrhea due to Abnormalities in the Hypothalamic-Pituitary-Ovarian Axis

Abnormality	Causes

Hypothalamic dysfunction	Functional hypothalamic amenorrhea
	    Weight loss, eating disorders
	    Exercise
	    Stress
	    Severe or prolonged illness
	Congenital gonadotropin-releasing hormone deficiency
	Inflammatory or infiltrative diseases
	Brain tumors - eg, craniopharyngioma
	Pituitary stalk dissection or compression
	Cranial irradiation
	Brain injury - trauma, hemorrhage, hydrocephalus
	Other syndromes - Prader-Willi, Laurence-Moon-Biedl

Pituitary dysfunction	Hyperprolactinemia Other pituitary tumors- acromegaly, corticotroph adenomas (Cushing's disease) Other tumors - meningioma, germinoma, glioma Empty sella syndrome Pituitary infarct or apoplexy

Ovarian dysfunction	Ovarian failure (menopause)
	    Spontaneous
	    Premature (before age 40 years)
	    Surgical

Other	Hyperthyroidism Hypothyroidism Diabetes mellitus Exogenous androgen use

Drugs Associated with Amenorrhea

Drugs that Increase Prolactin	Antipsychotics Tricyclic antidepressants Calcium channel blockers
Drugs with Estrogenic Activity	Digoxin, marijuana, oral contraceptives
Drugs with Ovarian Toxicity	Chemotherapeutic agents

C. **Step 3: Physical examination.** Measurements of height and weight, signs of other illnesses, and evidence of cachexia should be assessed. The skin, breasts, and genital tissues should be evaluated for estrogen deficiency. The breasts should be palpated, including an attempt to express galactorrhea. The skin should be examined for hirsutism, acne, striae, acanthosis nigricans, vitiligo, thickness or thinness, and easy bruisability.

D. **Step 4: Basic laboratory testing.** In addition to measurement of serum hCG to rule out pregnancy, minimal laboratory testing should include measurements of serum prolactin, thyrotropin, and FSH to rule out hyperprolactinemia, thyroid disease, and ovarian failure (high serum FSH). If there is hirsutism, acne or irregular menses, serum dehydroepiandrosterone sulfate (DHEA-S) and testosterone should be measured.

E. Step 5: Follow-up laboratory evaluation

1. **High serum prolactin concentration**. Prolactin secretion can be transiently increased by stress or eating. Therefore, serum prolactin should be measured at least twice before cranial imaging is obtained, particularly in those women with small elevations (<50 ng/mL). These women should be screened for thyroid disease with a TSH and free T4 because hypothyroidism can cause hyperprolactinemia.

2. Women with verified high serum prolactin values should have a cranial MRI unless a very clear explanation is found for the elevation (eg, antipsychotics). Imaging should rule out a hypothalamic or pituitary tumor.

3. **High serum FSH concentration**. A high serum FSH concentration indicates the presence of ovarian failure. This test should be repeated monthly on three occasions to confirm. A karyotype should be considered in most women with secondary amenorrhea age 30 years or younger.

4. **High serum androgen concentrations**. A high serum androgen value may suggest the diagnosis of polycystic ovary syndrome or may suggest an androgen-secreting tumor of the ovary or adrenal gland. Further testing for a tumor might include a 24-hour urine collection for cortisol and 17-ketosteroids, determination of serum 17-hydroxy-progesterone after intravenous injection of corticotropin (ACTH), and a dexamethasone suppression test. Elevation of 17-ketosteroids, DHEA-S, or 17-hydroxyprogesterone is more consistent with an adrenal, rather than ovarian, source of excess androgen.

5. **Normal or low serum gonadotropin concentrations and all other tests normal**
   a. This result is one of the most common outcomes of laboratory testing in women with amenorrhea. Women with hypothalamic amenorrhea (caused by marked exercise or weight loss to more than 10 percent below the expected weight) have normal to low serum FSH values. Cranial MRI is indicated in all women without an a clear explanation for hypogonadotropic hypogonadism and in most women who have visual field defects or headaches. No further testing is required if the onset of amenorrhea is recent or is easily explained (eg, weight loss, excessive exercise) and there are no symptoms suggestive of other disease.
   b. High serum transferrin saturation may indicate hemochromatosis, high serum angiotensin-converting enzyme values suggest sarcoidosis, and high fasting blood glucose or hemoglobin A1c values indicate diabetes mellitus.

6. **Normal serum prolactin and FSH concentrations with history of uterine instrumentation preceding amenorrhea**
   a. Evaluation for Asherman's syndrome should be completed. A progestin challenge should be performed (medroxyprogesterone acetate 10 mg for 10 days). If withdrawal bleeding occurs, an outflow tract disorder has been ruled out. If bleeding does not occur, estrogen and progestin should be administered.
   b. Oral conjugated estrogens (0.625 to 2.5 mg daily for 35 days) with medroxyprogesterone added (10 mg daily for days 26 to 35); failure to bleed upon cessation of this therapy strongly suggests endometrial scarring. In this situation, a hysterosalpingogram or hysteroscopy can confirm the diagnosis of Asherman syndrome.

II. Treatment

A. Athletic women should be counseled on the need for increased caloric intake or reduced exercise. Resumption of menses usually occurs.

B. Nonathletic women who are underweight should receive nutritional counseling and treatment of eating disorders.

C. Hyperprolactinemia is treated with a dopamine agonist. Cabergoline (Dostinex) or bromocriptine (Parlodel) are used for most adenomas.

Ovulation, regular menstrual cycles, and pregnancy may usually result.
- D. **Ovarian failure** should be treated with hormone replacement therapy.
- E. **Hyperandrogenism** is treated with measures to reduce hirsutism, resume menses, and fertility and preventing endometrial hyperplasia, obesity, and metabolic defects.
- F. **Asherman's syndrome** is treated with hysteroscopic lysis of adhesions followed by long-term estrogen administration to stimulate regrowth of endometrial tissue.

References: See page 166.

Menopause

Menopause is defined as the cessation of menstrual periods in women. The average age of menopause is 51 years, with a range of 41-55. The diagnosis of menopause is made by the presence of amenorrhea for six to twelve months, together with the occurrence of hot flashes. If the diagnosis is in doubt, menopause is indicated by an elevated follicle-stimulating hormone (FSH) level greater than 40 mIU/mL.

I. **Perimenopausal transition** is defined as the two to eight years preceding menopause and the one year after the last menstrual period. It is character-ized by normal ovulatory cycles interspersed with anovulatory (estrogen-only) cycles. As a result, menses become irregular, and heavy breakthrough bleeding, termed dysfunctional uterine bleeding, can occur during longer periods of anovulation.

II. **Effects of estrogen deficiency after menopause**
   - A. **Hot flashes.** The most common acute change during menopause is the hot flash, which occurs in 75 percent of women. About 50 to 75 percent of women have cessation of hot flashes within five years. Hot flashes typically begin as a sudden sensation of heat centered on the face and upper chest that rapidly becomes generalized. The sensation lasts from two to four minutes and is often associated with profuse perspiration. Hot flashes occur several times per day.
   - B. **Sexual function.** Estrogen deficiency leads to a decrease in blood flow to the vagina and vulva. This decrease is a major cause of decreased vaginal lubrication, dyspareunia, and decreased sexual function in menopausal women.
   - C. **Urinary incontinence.** Menopause results in atrophy of the urethral epithelium with subsequent atrophic urethritis and irritation; these changes predispose to both stress and urge urinary incontinence.
   - D. **Osteoporosis.** A long-term consequence of estrogen deficiency is the development of osteoporosis and fractures. Bone loss exceeds bone reformation. Between 1 and 5 percent of the skeletal mass can be lost per year in the first several years after the menopause. Osteoporosis may occur in as little as ten years.
   - E. **Cardiovascular disease.** The incidence of myocardial infarction in women, although lower than in men, increases dramatically after the menopause.

III. **Estrogen replacement therapy**
   - A. Data from the WHI and the HERS trials has determined that continuous estrogen-progestin therapy does not appear to protect against cardiovas-cular disease and increases the risk of breast cancer, coronary heart disease, stroke, and venous thromboembolism over an average follow-up of 5.2 years. As a result, the primary indication for estrogen therapy is for control of menopausal symptoms, such as hot flashes.

IV. **Prevention and treatment of osteoporosis**
   - A. **Screening for osteoporosis.** Measurement of BMD is recommended for all women 65 years and older regardless of risk factors. BMD should also be measured in all women under the age of 65 years who have one or more risk factors for osteoporosis (in addition to menopause). The hip is

the recommended site of measurement.

- **B. Bisphosphonates**
    1. **Alendronate (Fosamax)** has effects comparable to those of estrogen for both the treatment of osteoporosis (10 mg/day or 70 mg once a week) and for its prevention (5 mg/day). Alendronate (in a dose of 5 mg/day or 35 mg/week) can also prevent osteoporosis in postmenopausal women.
    2. **Risedronate (Actonel)**, a bisphosphonate, has been approved for prevention and treatment of osteoporosis at doses of 5 mg/day or 35 mg once per week. Its efficacy and side effect profile are similar to those of alendronate.
- **C. Raloxifene (Evista)** is a selective estrogen receptor modulator. It is available for prevention and treatment of osteoporosis. At a dose of 60 mg/day, bone density increases by 2.4 percent in the lumbar spine and hip over a two year period. This effect is slightly less than with bisphosphonates.
- **D. Calcium.** Maintaining a positive calcium balance in postmenopausal women requires a daily intake of 1500 mg of elemental calcium; to meet this most women require a supplement of 1000 mg daily.
- **E. Vitamin D.** All postmenopausal women should take a multivitamin containing at least 400 IU vitamin D daily.
- **F. Exercise** for at least 20 minutes daily reduces the rate of bone loss. Weight bearing exercises are preferable.
- **V. Treatment of hot flashes and vasomotor instability**
    - **A.** The manifestations of vasomotor instability are hot flashes, sleep disturbances, headache, and irritability. Most women with severe vasomotor instability accept short-term estrogen therapy for these symptoms.
    - **B. Short-term estrogen therapy for relief of vasomotor instability and hot flashes**
        1. Short-term estrogen therapy remains the best treatment for relief of menopausal symptoms, and therefore is recommended for most postmenopausal women, with the exception of those with a history of breast cancer, CHD, a previous venous thromboembolic event or stroke, or those at high risk for these complications. Short-term therapy is continued for six months to four or five years. Administration of estrogen short-term is not associated with an increased risk of breast cancer.
        2. Low dose estrogen is recommended (eg, 0.3 mg conjugated estrogens [Premarin] daily or 0.5 mg estradiol [Estrace] daily). These doses are adequate for symptom management and prevention of bone loss.
        3. Endometrial hyperplasia and cancer can occur after as little as six months of unopposed estrogen therapy; as a result, a progestin must be added in those women who have not had a hysterectomy. Medroxyprogesterone (Provera), 2.5 mg, is usually given every day of the month.
        4. After the planned treatment interval, the estrogen should be discontinued gradually to minimize recurrence of the menopausal symptoms, for example, by omitting one pill per week (6 pills per week, 5 pills per week, 4 pills per week).
    - **C. Treatment of vasomotor instability in women not taking estrogen**
        1. **Selective serotonin reuptake inhibitors** (SSRIs) also relieve the symptoms of vasomotor instability.
            - **a. Venlafaxine (Effexor)**, at doses of 75 mg daily, reduces hot flashes by 61 percent. Mouth dryness, anorexia, nausea, and constipation are common.
            - **b. Paroxetine (Zoloft)**, 50 mg per day, relieves vasomotor instability.
            - **c. Fluoxetine (Prozac)** 20 mg per day also has beneficial effects of a lesser magnitude.
        2. **Clonidine (Catapres)** relieves hot flashes in 80%. In a woman with hypertension, clonidine might be considered as initial therapy. It is

usually given as a patch containing 2.5 mg per week. Clonidine also may be given orally in doses of 0.1 to 0.4 mg daily. Side effects often limit the use and include dry mouth, dizziness, constipation, and sedation.

3. **Megestrol acetate (Megace)** is a synthetic progestin which decreases the frequency of hot flashes by 85 percent at a dose of 40 to 80 mg PO daily. Weight gain is the major side effect.

VI. **Treatment of urogenital atrophy**
   A. Loss of estrogen causes atrophy of the vaginal epithelium and results in vaginal irritation and dryness, dyspareunia, and an increase in vaginal infections. Systemic estrogen therapy results in relief of symptoms.
   B. **Treatment of urogenital atrophy in women not taking systemic estrogen**
      1. **Moisturizers and lubricants**. Regular use of a vaginal moisturizing agent (Replens) and lubricants during intercourse are helpful. Water soluble lubricants such as Astroglide are more effective than lubricants that become more viscous after application such as K-Y jelly. A more effective treatment is vaginal estrogen therapy.
      2. **Low-dose vaginal estrogen**
         a. **Vaginal ring estradiol (Estring)**, a silastic ring impregnated with estradiol, is the preferred means of delivering estrogen to the vagina. The silastic ring delivers 6 to 9 µg of estradiol to the vagina daily for a period of three months. The rings are changed once every three months by the patient. Concomitant progestin therapy is not necessary.
         b. **Conjugated estrogens (Premarin)**, 0.5 gm of cream, or one-eighth of an applicatorful daily into the vagina for three weeks, followed by twice weekly thereafter. Concomitant progestin therapy is not necessary.
         c. **Estrace cream (estradiol)** can also be given by vaginal applicator at a dose of one-eighth of an applicator or 0.5 g (which contains 50 µg of estradiol) daily into the vagina for three weeks, followed by twice weekly thereafter. Concomitant progestin therapy is not necessary.
         d. **Estradiol (Vagifem)**. A tablet containing 25 micrograms of estradiol is available and is inserted into the vagina twice per week. Concomitant progestin therapy is not necessary.

References: See page 166.

Premenstrual Syndrome and Premenstrual Dysphoric Disorder

Premenstrual syndrome (PMS) is characterized by physical and behavioral symptoms that occur repetitively in the second half of the menstrual cycle and interfere with some aspects of the woman's life. Premenstrual dysphoric disorder (PMDD) is the most severe form of PMS, with the prominence anger, irritability, and internal tension. PMS affects up to 75 percent of women with regular menstrual cycles, while PMDD affects only 3 to 8 percent of women.

I. **Symptoms**
   A. The most common physical manifestation of PMS is abdominal bloating, which occurs in 90 percent of women with this disorder; breast tenderness and headaches are also common, occurring in more than 50 percent of cases.
   B. The most common behavioral symptom of PMS is an extreme sense of fatigue which is seen in more than 90 percent. Other frequent behavioral complaints include irritability, tension, depressed mood, labile mood (80 percent), increased appetite (70 percent), and forgetfulness and difficulty concentrating (50 percent).
   C. Other common findings include acne, oversensitivity to environmental

stimuli, anger, easy crying, and gastrointestinal upset. Hot flashes, heart palpitations, and dizziness occur in 15 to 20 percent of patients. Symptoms should occur in the luteal phase only.

Symptom Clusters Commonly Noted in Patients with PMS

Affective Symptoms	**Cognitive or performance**
Depression or sadness	Mood instability or mood swings
Irritability	Difficulty in concentrating
Tension	Decreased efficiency
Anxiety	Confusion
Tearfulness or crying easily	Forgetfulness
Restlessness or jitteriness	Accident-prone
Anger	Social avoidance
Loneliness	Temper outbursts
Appetite change	Energetic
Food cravings	**Fluid retention**
Changes in sexual interest	Breast tenderness or swelling
Pain	Weight gain
Headache or migraine	Abdominal bloating or swelling
Back pain	Swelling of extremities
Breast pain	**General somatic**
Abdominal cramps	Fatigue or tiredness
General or muscular pain	Dizziness or vertigo
	Nausea
	Insomnia

DSM-IV Criteria for Premenstrual Dysphoric Disorder

- Five or more symptoms
- At least one of the following four symptoms:
  - Markedly depressed mood, feelings of hopelessness, or self-deprecating thoughts
  - Marked anxiety, tension, feeling of being "keyed up" or "on edge"
  - Marked affective lability
  - Persistent and marked anger or irritability or increase in interpersonal conflicts
- Additional symptoms that may be used to fulfill the criteria:
  - Decreased interest in usual activities
  - Subjective sense of difficulty in concentrating
  - Lethargy, easy fatigability, or marked lack of energy
  - Marked change in appetite, overeating, or specific food cravings
  - Hypersomnia or insomnia
  - Subjective sense of being overwhelmed or out of control
- Other physical symptoms such as breast tenderness or swelling, headaches, joint or muscle pain, a sensation of bloating, or weight gain
- Symptoms occurring during last week of luteal phase
- Symptoms are absent postmenstrually
- Disturbances that interfere with work or school or with usual social activities and relationships
- Disturbances that are not an exacerbation of symptoms of another disorder

---

D. DSM-IV criteria for premenstrual dysphoric disorder

1. Five or more of the following symptoms must have been present during the week prior to menses, resolving within a few days after menses starts. At least one of the five symptoms must be one of the first four on this list:
   a. Feeling sad, hopeless, or self-deprecating
   b. Feeling tense, anxious, or "on edge"
   c. Marked lability of mood interspersed with frequent tearfulness
   d. Persistent irritability, anger, and increased interpersonal conflicts
   e. Decreased interest in usual activities, which may be associated with withdrawal from social relationships
   f. Difficulty concentrating
   g. Feeling fatigued, lethargic, or lacking in energy

    h. Marked changes in appetite, which may be associated with binge eating or craving certain foods
    i. Hypersomnia or insomnia
    j. A subjective feeling of being overwhelmed or out of control
    k. Other physical symptoms, such as breast tenderness or swelling, headaches, joint or muscle pain, a sensation of bloating, weight gain.

UCSD Criteria for Premenstrual Syndrome

1. The presence by self report of at least one of the following somatic **and** affective symptoms during the five days prior to menses in each of the three menstrual cycles:

Affective	Somatic
Depression	Breast tenderness
Angry outbursts	Abdominal bloating
Irritability	Headache
Confusion	Swollen extremities
Social withdrawal	
Fatigue	

2. Relief of the above symptoms within four days of the onset of menses, without recurrence until at least cycle day 12.
3. The symptoms are present in the absence of any pharmacologic therapy, hormone ingestion, drug or alcohol use.
4. Identifiable dysfunction in social or economic performance by one of the following criteria:
    Marital or relationship discord confirmed by partner
    Difficulties in parenting
    Poor work or school performance, attendance/tardiness
    Increased social isolation
    Legal difficulties
    Suicidal Ideation
    Seeking medical attention for a somatic symptom(s)

  E. Differential diagnosis
    1. PMDD should be differentiated from premenstrual exacerbation of an underlying major psychiatric disorder, as well as medical conditions such as hyper- or hypothyroidism.
    2. About 13 percent of women with PMS are found to have a psychiatric disorder alone with no evidence of PMS, while 38 percent had premenstrual exacerbation of underlying depressive and anxiety disorders.
    3. Women who present with PMS have a much higher incidence of major depression in the past and are at greater risk for major depression in the future.
    4. 39 percent of women with PMDD meet criteria for mood or anxiety disorders.
    5. The assessment of patients with possible PMS or PMDD should begin with the history, physical examination, chemistry profile, complete blood count, and serum TSH. The history should focus in particular on the regularity of menstrual cycles. Appropriate gynecologic endocrine evaluation should be performed if the cycles are irregular (lengths less than 25 or greater than 36 days).
    6. The patient should be asked to record symptoms prospectively for two months. If the patient fails to demonstrate a symptom free interval in the follicular phase, she should be evaluated for a mood or anxiety disorder.

II. Treatment of premenstrual dysphoric disorder
  A. Serotonin reuptake inhibitors
    1. Fluoxetine (Sarafem) is an effective treatment for PMDD when given in a daily dose of 20 mg/day. The response rate is 60 to 75 percent. The most common reasons for failure to continue the treatment are headache, anxiety, and nausea.

    2. Other drugs that inhibit serotonin reuptake, such as clomipramine (Anafranil [given either throughout the menstrual cycle or restricted to the luteal phase]), sertraline (Zoloft) 50 to 150 mg/day throughout the menstrual cycle, and nefazodone (Serzone) 100-300 mg bid also may be effective in PMS.

    3. **Venlafaxine (Effexor)** selectively inhibits the reuptake of both serotonin and norepinephrine and is also effective (50 to 200 mg/day).

    4. Intermittent therapy given during the luteal phase only (starting on cycle day 14) has been shown to be effective.

B. Alprazolam (Xanax), 0.25 mg TID OR qid, has been shown in double-blind, placebo-controlled crossover studies to be beneficial in PMS.

C. GnRH agonists (leuprolide [Lupron] or buserelin) have shown some benefit. However, women with severe premenstrual depression are unresponsive to GnRH agonists. The physical symptoms may be more responsive than mood symptoms in women with PMS, and side effects (hypoestrogenism) may limit the use of these drugs for long-term therapy.

    1. **GnRH agonists and "add-back" therapy.** Add-back therapy with estrogen (and a progestin if indicated) mitigates concerns about bone loss from prolonged administration of GnRH agonists. Leuprolide alone led to a 75 percent improvement in luteal phase symptom scores. This benefit was maintained (60 percent improvement) during a crossover period in which estrogen/progestin replacement was added. Alendronate can be considered in women who do not tolerate hormonal add-back therapy but need osteoporosis prophylaxis.

D. Danazol inhibits pituitary gonadotropin secretion, and is an effective therapy for PMS. However, the androgenic side effects of danazol limit its use to patients who fail to respond adequately to the above therapies.

Treatment of Premenstrual Syndrome

Fluoxetine (Sarafem) 5-20 mg qd
Sertraline (Zoloft) 25-50 mg qd
Paroxetine (Paxil) 5-20 mg qd
Buspirone (BuSpar) 25 mg qd in divided doses

Alprazolam (Xanax) 0.25-0.50 mg tid

Mefenamic acid (Ponstel) 250 mg tid with meals

Other
Spirolactone (Aldactone) 25-200 mg qd
Cabergoline (Dostinex) 0.25 mg - 1 mg twice a week during the luteal phase for breast pain

---

E. Treatments with possible efficacy in PMS

    1. **Exercise and relaxation techniques.** There is suggestive evidence that exercise, relaxation, and reflexology may help to alleviate PMS symptoms.

    2. **Diuretics.** Spironolactone (Aldactone), 25-200 mg qd, may significantly decrease in negative mood symptom scores and somatic symptom.

F. Recommendations for the clinical management of PMS/PMDD

    1. Because of the proven efficacy and safety profile, serotonin reuptake inhibitors (SSRIs) are the first line therapy. Fluoxetine (Sarafem) has been the best studied. The effective dose is 20 mg/day.

    2. Approximately 15 percent of patients will experience significant side effects from an SSRI, including nausea, jitteryness, and headache. In such patients, a trial of either a lower starting dose or a second SSRI, such as sertraline (Zoloft) 25-50 mg qd, is warranted.

3. App...
   menst...
   (Xanax) ...
4. Patients wh...
   for ovulation s...
   GnRH agonists, t...
   attempt at "add-bac...

References: See page 166.

Abnormal Vaginal Bleedi...

Menorrhagia (excessive bleeding) is most co...
menstrual cycles. Occasionally it is caused by thyr...
cancer.

I. Pathophysiology of normal menstruation
   A. In response to gonadotropin-releasing hormone from t...
      the pituitary gland synthesizes follicle-stimulating hormo...
      luteinizing hormone (LH), which induce the ovaries to produ...
      and progesterone.
   B. During the follicular phase, estrogen stimulation causes an incre...
      endometrial thickness. After ovulation, progesterone causes endome...
      maturation. Menstruation is caused by estrogen and progesterone...
      withdrawal.
   C. **Abnormal bleeding** is defined as bleeding that occurs at intervals of less
      than 21 days, more than 36 days, lasting longer than 7 days, or blood loss
      greater than 80 mL.

II. Clinical evaluation of abnormal vaginal bleeding
   A. A menstrual and reproductive history should include last menstrual period,
      regularity, duration, frequency; the number of pads used per day, and
      intermenstrual bleeding.
   B. Stress, exercise, weight changes and systemic diseases, particularly
      thyroid, renal or hepatic diseases or coagulopathies, should be sought.
      The method of birth control should be determined.
   C. Pregnancy complications, such as spontaneous abortion, ectopic
      pregnancy, placenta previa and abruptio placentae, can cause heavy
      bleeding. Pregnancy should always be considered as a possible cause of
      abnormal vaginal bleeding.

III. Puberty and adolescence--menarche to age 16
   A. Irregularity is normal during the first few months of menstruation; however,
      soaking more than 25 pads or 30 tampons during a menstrual period is
      abnormal.
   B. Absence of premenstrual symptoms (breast tenderness, bloating,
      cramping) is associated with anovulatory cycles.
   C. Fever, particularly in association with pelvic or abdominal pain, may,
      indicate pelvic inflammatory disease. A history of easy bruising suggests
      a coagulation defect. Headaches and visual changes suggest a pituitary
      tumor.
   D. **Physical findings**
      1. Pallor not associated with tachycardia or signs of hypovolemia
         suggests chronic excessive blood loss secondary to anovulatory
         bleeding, adenomyosis, uterine myomas, or blood dyscrasia.
      2. Fever, leukocytosis, and pelvic tenderness suggests PID.
      3. Signs of impending shock indicate that the blood loss is related to
         pregnancy (including ectopic), trauma, sepsis, or neoplasia.
      4. Pelvic masses may represent pregnancy, uterine or ovarian neoplasia,
         or a pelvic abscess or hematoma.
      5. Fine, thinning hair, and hypoactive reflexes suggest hypothyroidism.
      6. Ecchymoses or multiple bruises may indicate trauma, coagulation
         defects, medication use, or dietary extremes.

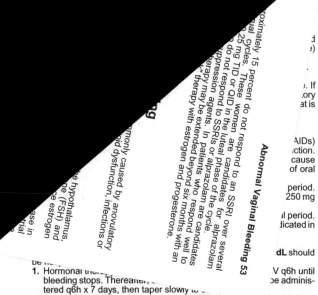

1. Hormonal ther... V q6h until bleeding stops. Thereafter, ... be administered q6h x 7 days, then taper slowly to ...
2. If bleeding continues, IV vasopressin (DDAVP) sh... be administered. Hysteroscopy may be necessary, and dilation and curettage is a last resort. Transfusion may be indicated in severe hemorrhage.
3. Iron should also be added as ferrous gluconate 325 mg tid.

IV. Primary childbearing years – ages 16 to early 40s

A. Contraceptive complications and pregnancy are the most common causes of abnormal bleeding in this age group. Anovulation accounts for 20% of cases.

B. Adenomyosis, endometriosis, and fibroids increase in frequency as a woman ages, as do endometrial hyperplasia and endometrial polyps. Pelvic inflammatory disease and endocrine dysfunction may also occur.

C. Laboratory tests
1. CBC and platelet count, Pap smear, and pregnancy test.
2. Screening for sexually transmitted diseases, thyroid-stimulating hormone, and coagulation disorders (partial thromboplastin time, INR, bleeding time).
3. If a non-pregnant woman has a pelvic mass, ultrasonography or hysterosonography (with uterine saline infusion) is required.

D. Endometrial sampling
1. Long-term unopposed estrogen stimulation in anovulatory patients can result in endometrial hyperplasia, which can progress to adeno-carcinoma; therefore, in perimenopausal patients who have been anovulatory for an extended interval, the endometrium should be biopsied.
2. Biopsy is also recommended before initiation of hormonal therapy for women over age 30 and for those over age 20 who have had prolonged bleeding.
3. Hysteroscopy and endometrial biopsy with a Pipelle aspirator should be done on the first day of menstruation (to avoid an unexpected pregnancy) or anytime if bleeding is continuous.

E. Treatment
  1. Medical protocols for anovulatory bleeding (dysfunctional uterine bleeding) are similar to those described above for adolescents.
  2. **Hormonal therapy**
      a. In women who do not desire immediate fertility, hormonal therapy may be used to treat menorrhagia.
      b. A 21-day package of oral contraceptives is used. The patient should take one pill three times a day for 7 days. During the 7 days of therapy, bleeding should subside, and, following treatment, heavy flow will occur. After 7 days off the hormones, another 21-day package is initiated, taking one pill each day for 21 days, then no pills for 7 days.
      c. Alternatively, medroxyprogesterone (Provera), 10-20 mg per day for days 16 through 25 of each month, will result in a reduction of menstrual blood loss. Pregnancy will not be prevented.
      d. Patients with severe bleeding may have hypotension and tachycardia. These patients require hospitalization, and estrogen (Premarin) should be administered IV as 25 mg q4-6h until bleeding slows (up to a maximum of four doses). Oral contraceptives should be initiated concurrently as described above.
  3. Iron should also be added as ferrous gluconate 325 mg tid.
  4. Surgical treatment can be considered if childbearing is completed and medical management fails to provide relief.

V. Premenopausal, perimenopausal, and postmenopausal years--age 40 and over
  A. Anovulatory bleeding accounts for about 90% of abnormal vaginal bleeding in this age group. However, bleeding should be considered to be from cancer until proven otherwise.
  B. History, physical examination and laboratory testing are indicated as described above. Menopausal symptoms, personal or family history of malignancy and use of estrogen should be sought. A pelvic mass requires an evaluation with ultrasonography.
  C. Endometrial carcinoma
  1. In a perimenopausal or postmenopausal woman, amenorrhea preceding abnormal bleeding suggests endometrial cancer. Endometrial evaluation is necessary before treatment of abnormal vaginal bleeding.
  2. Before endometrial sampling, determination of endometrial thickness by transvaginal ultrasonography is useful because biopsy is often not required when the endometrium is less than 5 mm thick.
  D. Treatment
  1. Cystic hyperplasia or endometrial hyperplasia without cytologic atypia is treated with depo-medroxyprogesterone, 200 mg IM, then 100 to 200 mg IM every 3 to 4 weeks for 6 to 12 months. Endometrial hyperplasia requires repeat endometrial biopsy every 3 to 6 months.
  2. Atypical hyperplasia requires fractional dilation and curettage, followed by progestin therapy or hysterectomy.
  3. If the patient's endometrium is normal (or atrophic) and contraception is a concern, a low-dose oral contraceptive may be used. If contraception is not needed, estrogen and progesterone therapy should be prescribed.
  4. **Surgical management**
      a. **Vaginal or abdominal hysterectomy** is the most absolute curative treatment.
      b. **Dilatation and curettage** can be used as a temporizing measure to stop bleeding.
      c. **Endometrial ablation and resection** by laser, electrodiathermy "rollerball," or excisional resection are alternatives to hysterectomy.

References: See page 166.

Breast Cancer Screening and Diagnosis

Breast cancer is the most common form of cancer in women. There are 200,000 new cases of breast cancer each year, resulting in 47,000 deaths per year. The lifetime risk of breast cancer is one in eight for a woman who is age 20. For patients under age 60, the chance of being diagnosed with breast cancer is 1 in about 400 in a given year.

I. Pathophysiology

A. The etiology of breast cancer remains unknown, but two breast cancer genes have been cloned–the BRCA-1 and the BRCA-2 genes. Only 10% of all of the breast cancers can be explained by mutations in these genes.

B. Estrogen stimulation is an important promoter of breast cancer, and, therefore, patients who have a long history of menstruation are at increased risk. Early menarche and late menopause are risk factors for breast cancer. Late age at birth of first child or nulliparity also increase the risk of breast cancer.

C. Family history of breast cancer in a first degree relative and history of benign breast disease also increase the risk of breast cancer. The use of estrogen replacement therapy or oral contraceptives slightly increases the risk of breast cancer. Radiation exposure and alcoholic beverage consumption also increase the risk of breast cancer.

Recommended Intervals for Breast Cancer Screening Studies			
	Age <40 yr	40-49 yr	50-75 yr
Breast Self-Examination	Monthly by age 30	Monthly	Monthly
Professional Breast Examination	Every 3 yr, ages 20-39	Annually	Annually
Mammography, Low Risk Patient		Annually	Annually
Mammography, High Risk Patient	Begin at 35 yr	Annually	Annually

II. Diagnosis and evaluation

A. **Clinical evaluation of a breast mass** should assess duration of the lesion, associated pain, relationship to the menstrual cycle or exogenous hormone use, and change in size since discovery. The presence of nipple discharge and its character (bloody or tea-colored, unilateral or bilateral, spontaneous or expressed) should be assessed.

B. **Menstrual history.** The date of last menstrual period, age of menarche, age of menopause or surgical removal of the ovaries, regularity of the menstrual cycle, previous pregnancies, age at first pregnancy, and lactation history should be determined.

C. **History of previous breast biopsies,** breast cancer, or cyst aspiration should be investigated. Previous or current oral contraceptive and hormone replacement therapy and dates and results of previous mammograms should be ascertained.

D. **Family history** should document breast cancer in relatives and the age at which family members were diagnosed.

III. Physical examination

A. The breasts should be inspected for asymmetry, deformity, skin retraction, erythema, peau d'orange (indicating breast edema), and nipple retraction, discoloration, or inversion.

B. Palpation
1. The breasts should be palpated while the patient is sitting and then supine with the ipsilateral arm extended. The entire breast should be palpated systematically.
2. The mass should be evaluated for size, shape, texture, tenderness, fixation to skin or chest wall. The location of the mass should be documented with a diagram in the patient's chart. The nipples should be expressed to determine whether discharge can be induced. Nipple discharge should be evaluated for single or multiple ducts, color, and any associated mass.
3. The axillae should be palpated for adenopathy, with an assessment of size of the lymph nodes, their number, and fixation. The supraclavicular and cervical nodes should also be assessed.

IV. Breast imaging
A. Mammography
1. **Screening mammography** is performed in the asymptomatic patients and consists of two views. Patients are not examined by a mammographer. Screening mammography reduces mortality from breast cancer and should usually be initiated at age 40.
2. **Diagnostic mammography** is performed after a breast mass has been detected. Patients usually are examined by a mammographer, and films are interpreted immediately and additional views of the lesion are completed. Mammographic findings predictive of malignancy include spiculated masses with architectural distortion and microcalcifications. A normal mammography in the presence of a palpable mass does not exclude malignancy.

B. Ultrasonography is used as an adjunct to mammography to differentiate solid from cystic masses. It is the primary imaging modality in patients younger than 30 years old.

V. Methods of breast biopsy
A. Stereotactic core needle biopsy. Using a computer-driven stereotactic unit, the lesion is localized in three dimensions, and an automated biopsy needle obtains samples. The sensitivity and specificity of this technique are 95-100% and 94-98%, respectively.

B. Palpable masses. Fine-needle aspiration biopsy (FNAB) has a sensitivity ranging from 90-98%. Nondiagnostic aspirates require surgical biopsy.
1. The skin is prepped with alcohol and the lesion is immobilized with the nonoperating hand. A 10 mL syringe, with a 18 to 22 gauge needle, is introduced in to the central portion of the mass at a 90° angle. When the needle enters the mass, suction is applied by retracting the plunger, and the needle is advanced. The needle is directed into different areas of the mass while maintaining suction on the syringe.
2. Suction is slowly released before the needle is withdrawn from the mass. The contents of the needle are placed onto glass slides for pathologic examination.

C. Impalpable lesions
1. **Needle localized biopsy**
   a. Under mammographic guidance, a needle and hookwire are placed into the breast parenchyma adjacent to the lesion. The patient is taken to the operating room along with mammograms for an excisional breast biopsy.
   b. The skin and underlying tissues are infiltrated with 1% lidocaine with epinephrine. For lesions located within 5 cm of the nipple, a periareolar incision may be used or use a curved incision located over the mass and parallel to the areola. Incise the skin and subcutaneous fat, then palpate the lesion and excise the mass.
   c. After removal of the specimen, a specimen x-ray is performed to confirm that the lesion has been removed. The specimen can then be sent fresh for pathologic analysis.

        d. Close the subcutaneous tissues with a 4-0 chromic catgut suture, and close the skin with 4-0 subcuticular suture.

References: See page 166.

Breast Disorders

Breast pain, nipple discharge and a palpable mass are the most common breast problems for which women consult a physician.

I. Nipple Discharge
A. Clinical evaluation
    1. Nipple discharge may be a sign of cancer; therefore, it must be thoroughly evaluated. About 8% of biopsies performed for nipple discharge demonstrate cancer. The duration, bilaterality or unilaterality of the discharge, and the presence of blood should be determined. A history of oral contraceptives, hormone preparations, phenothiazines, nipple or breast stimulation or lactation should be sought. Discharges that flow spontaneously are more likely to be pathologic than discharges that must be manually expressed.

    2. Unilateral, pink colored, bloody or non-milky discharge, or discharges associated with a mass are the discharges of most concern. Milky discharge can be caused by oral contraceptive agents, estrogen replacement therapy, phenothiazines, prolactinoma, or hypothyroidism. Nipple discharge secondary to malignancy is more likely to occur in older patients.

    3. **Risk factors.** The assessment should identify risk factors, including age over 50 years, past personal history of breast cancer, history of hyperplasia on previous breast biopsies, and family history of breast cancer in a first-degree relative (mother, sister, daughter).

B. Physical examination should include inspection of the breast for ulceration or contour changes and inspection of the nipple. Palpation should be performed with the patient in both the upright and the supine positions to determine the presence of a mass.

C. Diagnostic evaluation
    1. **Bloody discharge.** A mammogram of the involved breast should be obtained if the patient is over 35 years old and has not had a mammogram within the preceding 6 months. Biopsy of any suspicious lesions should be completed.

    2. **Watery, unilateral discharge** should be referred to a surgeon for evaluation and possible biopsy.

    3. **Non-bloody discharge** should be tested for the presence of blood with a Hemoccult card. Nipple discharge secondary to carcinoma usually contains hemoglobin.

    4. **Milky, bilateral discharge** should be evaluated with assays of prolactin and thyroid stimulating hormone to exclude an endocrinologic cause.
        a. A mammogram should be performed if the patient is due for routine mammographic screening.
        b. If results of the mammogram and the endocrinologic screening studies are normal, the patient should return for a follow-up visit in 6 months to ensure that there has been no specific change in the character of the discharge, such as development of bleeding.

II. Breast Pain
A. Breast pain is the most common breast symptom causing women to consult primary care physicians. Mastalgia is more common in premenopausal women than in postmenopausal women, and it is rarely a presenting symptom of breast cancer.

B. The evaluation of breast pain should determine the type of pain, its location and its relationship to the menstrual cycle. Most commonly, breast pain is associated with the menstrual cycle (cyclic mastalgia).

C. Cyclic pain is usually bilateral and poorly localized. The pain is often relieved after the menses. Cyclic breast pain occurs more often in younger women and resolves spontaneously.

D. Noncyclic mastalgia is most common in women 40 to 50 years of age. It is often a unilateral pain. Noncyclic mastalgia is occasionally secondary to the presence of a fibroadenoma or cyst, and the pain may be relieved by treatment of the underlying breast lesion.

E. **Evaluation.** A thorough breast examination should be performed to exclude the presence of a breast mass. Women 35 years of age and older should undergo mammography unless a mammogram was obtained in the past 12 months. If a suspicious lesion is detected, biopsy is required. When the physical examination is normal, imaging studies are not indicated in women younger than 35 years of age. A follow-up clinical breast examination should be performed in 1-2 months.

F. **Mastodynia**
   1. Mastodynia is defined as breast pain in the absence of a mass or other pathologic abnormality.
   2. **Causes of mastodynia** include menstrually related pain, costochondritis, trauma, and sclerosing adenosis.

III. **Fibrocystic Complex**
   A. Breast changes are usually multifocal, bilateral, and diffuse. One or more isolated fibrocystic lumps or areas of asymmetry may be present. The areas are usually tender.
   B. This disorder predominantly occurs in women with premenstrual abnormalities, nulliparous women, and nonusers of oral contraceptives.
   C. The disorder usually begins in mid-20's or early 30's. Tenderness is associated with menses and lasts about a week. The upper outer quadrant of the breast is most frequently involved bilaterally. There is no increased risk of cancer for the majority of patients.
   D. Suspicious areas may be evaluated by fine needle aspiration (FNA) cytology. If mammography and FNA are negative for cancer, and the clinical examination is benign, open biopsy is generally not needed.
   E. **Medical management of fibrocystic complex**
      1. **Oral contraceptives** are effective for severe breast pain in most young women. Start with a pill that contains low amounts of estrogen and relatively high amounts of progesterone (Loestrin, LoOvral, Ortho-Cept).
      2. If oral contraceptives do not provide relief, medroxyprogesterone, 5-10 mg/day from days 15-25 of each cycle, is added.
      3. A professionally fitted support bra often provides significant relief.
      4. **Danazol (Danocrine),** an antigonadotropin, has a response rate of 50 to 75 percent in women with cyclic pain who received danazol in a dosage of 100 to 400 mg per day. Danazol therapy is recommended only for patients with severe, activity-limiting pain. Side effects include menstrual irregularity, acne, weight gain and hirsutism.
      5. **Evening primrose oil** (g-linolenic acid) is effective in about 38 to 58 percent of patients with mastalgia; 2 - 4 g per day.

IV. **Breast Masses**
   A. The normal glandular tissue of the breast is nodular. Nodularity is a physiologic process and is not an indication of breast pathology. Dominant masses may be discrete or poorly defined, but they differ in character from the surrounding breast tissue. The differential diagnosis of a dominant breast mass includes macrocyst (clinically evident cyst), fibroadenoma, prominent areas of fibrocystic change, fat necrosis and cancer.
   B. **Cystic Breast Masses**
      1. Cysts are a common cause of dominant breast masses in premenopausal women more than 40 years of age, but they are an infrequent cause of such masses in younger women. Cysts are usually well demarcated, firm and mobile.
      2. Ultrasonography or aspiration must establish a definitive diagnosis for a cyst. Cysts require surgical biopsy if the aspirated fluid is bloody, the palpable abnormality does not resolve completely after the aspiration

of fluid or the same cyst recurs multiple times in a short period of time. Routine cytologic examination of cyst fluid is not indicated.

3. **Nonpalpable cysts** identified by mammography and confirmed to be simple cysts by ultrasound examination require no treatment.

C. **Solid Breast Masses**

1. Noncystic masses in premenopausal women that are clearly different from the surrounding breast tissue require histologic sampling by fine-needle aspiration, core cutting, needle biopsy or excisional biopsy.

2. **Solid Masses in Women Less Than 40 Years of Age**
   a. If the physical examination reveals no evidence of a dominant breast mass, the patient should be reassured and instructed in breast self-examination. If the clinical significance of a physical finding is uncertain, a directed ultrasound examination is performed. If this examination does not demonstrate a mass, the physical examination is repeated in two to four months. In women 35 to 40 years of age who have a normal ultrasound examination, a mammogram may also be obtained.
   b. A suspicious mass is solitary, discrete, hard and adherent to adjacent tissue. Mammography should be performed before obtaining a pathologic diagnosis.
   c. If a clinically benign mass is present, an ultrasound examination and fine-needle aspiration are performed to confirm that the mass is benign. This approach is the "triple test" (clinical examination, ultra-sonography [or mammography] and fine-needle aspiration).

3. **Solid Masses in Women More Than 40 Years of Age.** Abnormalities detected on physical examination in older women should be regarded as possible cancers until they are proven to be benign. In women more than 40 years of age, diagnostic mammography is a standard part of the evaluation of a solid breast mass.

References: See page 166.

Sexual Assault

Sexual assault is defined as any sexual act performed by one person on another without the person's consent. Sexual assault includes genital, anal, or oral penetration by a part of the accused's body or by an object. It may result from force, the threat of force, or the victim's inability to give consent. The annual incidence of sexual assault is 200 per 100,000 persons.

I. **Psychological effects**
   A. A woman who is sexually assaulted loses control over her life during the period of the assault. Her integrity and her life are threatened. She may experience intense anxiety, anger, or fear. After the assault, a "rape-trauma" syndrome often occurs. The immediate response may last for hours or days and is characterized by generalized pain, headache, chronic pelvic pain, eating and sleep disturbances, vaginal symptoms, depression, anxiety, and mood swings.
   B. The delayed phase is characterized by flashbacks, nightmares, and phobias.

II. **Medical evaluation**
   A. Informed consent must be obtained before the examination. Acute injuries should be stabilized. About 1% of injuries require hospitalization and major operative repair, and 0.1% of injuries are fatal.
   B. A history and physical examination should be performed. A chaperon should be present during the history and physical examination to reassure the victim and provide support. The patient should be asked to state in her own words what happened, identify her attacker if possible, and provide details of the act(s) performed if possible.

Clinical Care of the Sexual Assault Victim

Medical
Obtain informed consent from the patient
Obtain a gynecologic history
Assess and treat physical injuries
Obtain appropriate cultures and treat any existing infections
Provide prophylactic antibiotic therapy and offer immunizations
Provide therapy to prevent unwanted conception
Offer baseline serologic tests for hepatitis B virus, human immunodeficiency virus (HIV), and syphilis
Provide counseling
Arrange for follow-up medical care and counseling

Legal
Provide accurate recording of events
Document injuries
Collect samples (pubic hair, fingernail scrapings, vaginal secretions, saliva, blood-stained clothing)
Report to authorities as required
Assure chain of evidence

C. Previous obstetric and gynecologic conditions should be sought, particularly infections, pregnancy, use of contraception, and date of the last menstrual period. Preexisting pregnancy, risk for pregnancy, and the possibility of preexisting infections should be assessed.

D. **Physical examination** of the entire body and photographs or drawings of the injured areas should be completed. Bruises, abrasions, and lacerations should be sought. Superficial or extensive lacerations of the hymen and vagina, injury to the urethra, and occasionally rupture of the vaginal vault into the abdominal cavity may be noted. Bite marks are common.

   1. **Pelvic examination** should assess the status of the reproductive organs, collect samples from the cervix and vagina, and test for Neisseria gonorrhoeae and Chlamydia trachomatis.

   2. **A Wood light** should be used to find semen on the patient's body: dried semen will fluoresce. Sperm and other Y-chromosome-bearing cells may be identified from materials collected from victims.

E. **A serum sample** should be obtained for baseline serology for syphilis, herpes simplex virus, hepatitis B virus, and HIV.

F. **Trichomonas** is the most frequently acquired STD. The risk of acquiring human immunodeficiency virus (HIV) <1% during a single act of heterosexual intercourse, but the risk depends on the population involved and the sexual acts performed. The risk of acquiring gonorrhea is 6-12%, and the risk of acquiring syphilis is 3%.

G. **Hepatitis B virus** is 20 times more infectious than HIV during sexual intercourse. Hepatitis B immune globulin (0.06 mL of hepatitis B immune globulin per kilogram) should be administered intramuscularly as soon as possible within 14 days of exposure. It is followed by the standard three-dose immunization series with hepatitis B vaccine (0, 1, and 6 months), beginning at the time of hepatitis B immune globulin administration.

H. **Emergency contraception.** If the patient is found to be at risk for pregnancy as a result of the assault, emergency contraception should be offered. The risk of pregnancy after sexual assault is 2-4% in victims not already using contraception. One dose of combination oral contraceptive tablets is given at the time the victim is seen and an additional dose is given in 12 hours. Emergency contraception can be effective up to 120 hours after unprotected coitus. Metoclopramide (Reglan), 20 mg with each dose of hormone, is prescribed for nausea. A pregnancy test should be performed at the 2-week return visit if conception is suspected.

Emergency Contraception

1. Consider pretreatment one hour before each oral contraceptive pill dose, using one of the following orally administered antiemetic agents:
   Prochlorperazine (Compazine), 5 to 10 mg
   Promethazine (Phenergan), 12.5 to 25 mg
   Trimethobenzamide (Tigan), 250 mg
2. Administer the first dose of oral contraceptive pill within 72 hours of intercourse, and administer the second dose 12 hours after the first dose. Brand name options for emergency contraception include the following:
   Preven Kit--two pills per dose (0.5 mg of levonorgestrel and 100 µg of ethinyl estradiol per dose)
   Ovral--two pills per dose (0.5 mg of levonorgestrel and 100 µg of ethinyl estradiol per dose)
   Plan B--one pill per dose (0.75 mg of levonorgestrel per dose)
   Nordette--four pills per dose (0.6 mg of levonorgestrel and 120 µg of ethinyl estradiol per dose)
   Triphasil--four pills per dose (0.5 mg of levonorgestrel and 120 µg of ethinyl estradiol per dose)

Screening and Treatment of Sexually Transmissible Infections Following Sexual Assault

Initial Examination

Infection
- Testing for and gonorrhea and chlamydia from specimens from any sites of penetration or attempted penetration
- Wet mount and culture or a vaginal swab specimen for Trichomonas
- Serum sample for syphilis, herpes simplex virus, hepatitis B virus, and HIV

Pregnancy Prevention

Prophylaxis
- Hepatitis B virus vaccination and hepatitis B immune globulin.
- Empiric recommended antimicrobial therapy for chlamydial, gonococcal, and trichomonal infections and for bacterial vaginosis:
  Ceftriaxone, 125 mg intramuscularly in a single dose, plus
  Metronidazole, 2 g orally in a single dose, plus
  Doxycycline 100 mg orally two times a day for 7 days
  Azithromycin (Zithromax) is used if the patient is unlikely to comply with the 7 day course of doxycycline; single dose of four 250 mg caps.
  If the patient is penicillin-allergic, ciprofloxacin 500 mg PO or ofloxacin 400 mg PO is substituted for ceftriaxone. If the patient is pregnant, erythromycin 500 mg PO qid for 7 days is substituted for doxycycline.
  HIV prophylaxis consists of zidovudine (AZT) 200 mg PO tid, plus lamivudine (3TC) 150 mg PO bid for 4 weeks.

Follow-Up Examination (2 weeks)

- Cultures for N gonorrhoeae and C trachomatis (not needed if prophylactic treatment has been provided)
- Wet mount and culture for T vaginalis
- Collection of serum sample for subsequent serologic analysis if test results are positive

Follow-Up Examination (12 weeks)

Serologic tests for infectious agents:
   T pallidum
   HIV (repeat test at 6 months)
   Hepatitis B virus (not needed if hepatitis B virus vaccine was given)

III. **Emotional care**
   A. The physician should discuss the injuries and the probability of infection or pregnancy with the victim, and she should be allowed to express her anxieties.
   B. Anxiolytic medication may be useful; lorazepam (Ativan) 1-5 mg PO tid prn anxiety.
   C. The patient should be referred to personnel trained to handle rape-trauma victims within 1 week.
IV. **Follow-up care**
   A. The patient is seen for medical follow-up in 2 weeks for documentation of healing of injuries.
   B. Repeat testing includes syphilis, hepatitis B, and gonorrhea and chlamydia cultures. HIV serology should be repeated in 3 months and 6 months.
   C. A pregnancy test should be performed if conception is suspected.
References: See page 166.

Osteoporosis

Over 1.3 million osteoporotic fractures occur each year in the United States. The risk of all fractures increases with age; among persons who survive until age 90, 33 percent of women will have a hip fracture. The lifetime risk of hip fracture for white women at age 50 is 16 percent. Osteoporosis is characterized by low bone mass, microarchitectural disruption, and increased skeletal fragility.

Risk Factors for Osteoporotic Fractures	
Personal history of fracture as an adult History of fracture in a first-degree relative Current cigarette smoking Low body weight (less than 58 kg [127 lb]) Female sex Estrogen deficiency (menopause before age 45 years or bilateral ovariectomy, prolonged premenopausal amenorrhea [greater than one year])	White race Advanced age Lifelong low calcium intake Alcoholism Inadequate physical activity Recurrent falls Dementia Impaired eyesight despite adequate correction Poor health/frailty

I. **Screening for osteoporosis and osteopenia**
   A. **Normal bone density** is defined as a bone mineral density (BMD) value within one standard deviation of the mean value in young adults of the same sex and race.
   B. **Osteopenia** is defined as a BMD between 1 and 2.5 standard deviations below the mean.
   C. **Osteoporosis** is defined as a value more than 2.5 standard deviations below the mean; this level is the fracture threshold. These values are referred to as T-scores (number of standard deviations above or below the mean value).
   D. **Dual x-ray absorptiometry.** In dual x-ray absorptiometry (DXA), two photons are emitted from an x-ray tube. DXA is the most commonly used

method for measuring bone density because it gives very precise measurements with minimal radiation. DXA measurements of the spine and hip are recommended.

E. **Biochemical markers of bone turnover. Urinary deoxypyridinoline (DPD) and urinary alpha-1 to alpha-2 N-telopeptide of collagen (NTX)** are the most specific and clinically useful markers of bone resorption. Biochemical markers are not useful for the screening or diagnosis of osteoporosis because the values in normal and osteoporosis overlap substantially.

II. **Recommendations for screening for oseteoporosis of the National Osteoporosis Foundation**

A. All women should be counseled about the risk factors for osteoporosis, especially smoking cessation and limiting alcohol. All women should be encouraged to participate in regular weight-bearing and exercise.

B. Measurement of BMD is recommended for all women 65 years and older regardless of risk factors. BMD should also be measured in all women under the age of 65 years who have one or more risk factors for osteoporosis (in addition to menopause). The hip is the recommended site of measurement.

C. All adults should be advised to consume at least 1,200 mg of calcium per day and 400 to 800 IU of vitamin D per day. A daily multivitamin (which provides 400 IU) is recommended. In patients with documented vitamin D deficiency, osteoporosis, or previous fracture, two multivitamins may be reasonable, particularly if dietary intake is inadequate and access to sunlight is poor.

D. Treatment is recommended for women without risk factors who have a BMD that is 2 SD below the mean for young women, and in women with risk factors who have a BMD that is 1.5 SD below the mean.

III. **Nonpharmacologic therapy of osteoporosis in women**

A. **Diet.** An optimal diet for treatment (or prevention) of osteoporosis includes an adequate intake of calories (to avoid malnutrition), calcium, and vitamin D.

B. **Calcium.** Postmenopausal women should be advised to take 1000 to 1500 mg/day of elemental calcium, in divided doses, with meals.

C. **Vitamin D** total of 800 IU daily should be taken.

D. **Exercise.** Women should exercise for at least 30 minutes three times per week. Any weight-bearing exercise regimen, including walking, is acceptable.

E. **Cessation of smoking** is recommended for all women because smoking cigarettes accelerates bone loss.

IV. **Drug therapy of osteoporosis in women**

A. Selected postmenopausal women with osteoporosis or at high risk for the disease should be considered for drug therapy. Particular attention should be paid to treating women with a recent fragility fracture, including hip fracture, because they are at high risk for a second fracture.

B. Candidates for drug therapy are women who already have postmenopausal osteoporosis (less than -2.5) and women with osteopenia (T score -1 to -2.5) soon after menopause.

C. **Bisphosphonates**

1. **Alendronate (Fosamax)** (10 mg/day or 70 mg once weekly) or **risedronate (Actonel)** (5 mg/day or 35 mg once weekly) are good choices for the treatment of osteoporosis. Bisphosphonate therapy increases bone mass and reduces the incidence of vertebral and nonvertebral fractures.

2. Alendronate (5 mg/day or 35 mg once weekly) and risedronate (5 mg/day of 35 mg once weekly) have been approved for prevention of osteoporosis.

3. Alendronate or risedronate should be taken with a full glass of water 30 minutes before the first meal or beverage of the day. Patients should not lie down for at least 30 minutes after taking the dose to avoid the unusual complication of pill-induced esophagitis.

4. Alendronate is well tolerated and effective for at least seven years.

5. The bisphosphonates (alendronate or risedronate) and raloxifene are first-line treatments for *prevention* of osteoporosis. The bisphosphonates are first-line therapy for *treatment* of osteoporosis. Bisphosphonates are preferred for prevention and treatment of osteoporosis because they increase bone mineral density more than raloxifene.

D. Selective estrogen receptor modulators

1. **Raloxifene (Evista)** (5 mg daily or a once-a-week preparation) is a selective estrogen receptor modulator (SERM) for prevention and treatment of osteoporosis. It increases bone mineral density and reduces serum total and low-density-lipoprotein (LDL) cholesterol. It also appears to reduce the incidence of vertebral fractures and is one of the first-line drugs for prevention of osteoporosis.

2. Raloxifene is somewhat less effective than the bisphosphonates for the prevention and treatment of osteoporosis. Venous thromboembolism is a risk.

Treatment Guidelines for Osteoporosis

Calcium supplements with or without vitamin D supplements or calcium-rich diet
Weight-bearing exercise
Avoidance of alcohol tobacco products
Alendronate (Fosamax)
Risedronate (Actonel)
Raloxifene (Evista)

Agents for Treating Osteoporosis

Medication	Dosage	Route
Calcium	1,000 to 1,500 mg per day	Oral
Vitamin D	400 IU per day (800 IU per day in winter in northern latitudes)	Oral
Alendronate (Fosamax)	**Prevention:** 5 mg per day or 35 mg once-a-week **Treatment:** 10 mg per day or 70 mg once-a-week	Oral
Risedronate (Actonel)	5 mg daily or 35 mg once weekly	Oral
Raloxifene (Evista)	60 mg per day	Oral
Conjugated estrogens	0.3 mg per day	Oral

E. Monitoring the response to therapy

1. Bone mineral density and a marker of bone turnover should be measured at baseline, followed by a repeat measurement of the marker in three months.

2. If the marker falls appropriately, the drug is having the desired effect, and therapy should be continued for two years, at which time bone mineral density can be measured again. The anticipated three-month decline in markers is 50 percent with alendronate.

F. **Estrogen/progestin therapy**
1. Estrogen-progestin therapy is no longer a first-line approach for the treatment of osteoporosis in postmenopausal women because of increases in the risk of breast cancer, stroke, venous thrombo-embolism, and coronary disease.
2. Indications for estrogen-progestin in postmenopausal women include persistent menopausal symptoms and patients with an indication for antiresorptive therapy who cannot tolerate the other drugs.

References: See page 166.

Infertility

Infertility is defined as failure of a couple of reproductive age to conceive after 12 months or more of regular coitus without using contraception. Infertility is considered primary when it occurs in a woman who has never established a pregnancy and secondary when it occurs in a woman who has a history of one or more previous pregnancies. Fecundability is defined as the probability of achieving a pregnancy within one menstrual cycle. It is estimated that 10% to 20% of couples are infertile.

I. **Diagnostic evaluation**
  A. **History**
  1. The history should include the couple's ages, the duration of infertility, previous infertility in other relationships, frequency of coitus, and use of lubricants (which can be spermicidal). Mumps orchitis, renal disease, radiation therapy, sexually transmitted diseases, chronic disease such as tuberculosis, major stress and fatigue, or a recent history of acute viral or febrile illness should be sought. Exposure to radiation, chemicals, excessive heat from saunas or hot tubs should be investigated.
  2. Pelvic inflammatory disease, previous pregnancies, douching practices, work exposures, alcohol and drug use, exercise, and history of any eating disorders should be evaluated.
  3. Menstrual cycle length and regularity and indirect indicators of ovulation, such as Mittelschmerz, mid-cycle cervical mucus change and premenstrual molimina, should be assessed.
  B. **Physical examination for the woman**
  1. Vital signs, height, and weight should be noted. Hypertension hair distribution, acne, hirsutism, thyromegaly, enlarged lymph nodes, abdominal masses or scars, galactorrhea, or acanthosis nigricans (suggestive of diabetes) should be sought.
  2. Pelvic examination should include a Papanicolaou smear and bimanual examination to assess uterine size and any ovarian masses.
  3. Testing for Chlamydia trachomatis, Mycoplasma hominis, and Ureaplasma urealyticum are recommended.
  C. **Physical examination for the man**
  1. Height, weight, and hair distribution, gynecomastia, palpable lymph nodes or thyromegaly should be sought.
  2. The consistency, size, and position of both testicles and the presence of varicocele or abnormal location of the urethral meatus on the penis should be noted. Testing for Chlamydia, Ureaplasma, and Mycoplasma should be completed.
  D. The cornerstone of any infertility evaluation relies on the assessment of six basic elements: (1) semen analysis, (2) sperm-cervical mucus interaction, (3) ovulation, (4) tubal patency, and (5) uterine and (6) peritoneal abnormalities. Couples of reproductive age who have intercourse regularly without contraception have approximately a 25-30% chance of conceiving in a given menstrual cycle and an 85% chance of conceiving within 1 year.
  E. **Semen analysis.** The specimen is routinely obtained by masturbation

and collected in a clean glass or plastic container. It is customary to have the man abstain from ejaculation for at least 2 days before producing the specimen. Criteria for a normal semen analysis include a sperm count greater than 20 million sperm/mL with at least 50% motility and 30% normal morphology.

Semen Analysis Interpretation		
Semen Parameter	**Normal Values**	**Poor Prognosis**
Sperm concentration	>20 x 106/mL	<5 million/ mL
Sperm motility	>50% progressive motility	<10% motility
Sperm morphology	>50% normal	<4% normal
Ejaculate volume	>2 cc	<2 cc

F. The postcoital test (PCT) is used to assess sperm-cervical mucus interaction after intercourse. The PCT provides information regarding cervical mucus quality and survivability of sperm after intercourse. The PCT should be performed 8 hours after intercourse and 1 to 2 days before the predicted time of ovulation, when there is maximum estrogen secretion unopposed by progesterone.

G. Ovulation assessment

1. Commonly used methods used to assess ovulation include measuring a rise in basal body temperature (BBT), identifying an elevation in the midluteal phase serum progesterone concentration, luteal phase endometrial biopsy, and detection of luteinizing hormone (LH) in the urine. The BBT chart is used to acquire information regarding ovulation and the duration of the luteal phase. Female patients are instructed to take their temperature upon awaking each morning before any physical activity. A temperature rise of 0.4°F (0.22°C) for 2 consecutive days is indicative of ovulation. The initial rise in serum progesterone level occurs between 48 hours before ovulation and 24 hours after ovulation. For this reason, a rise in temperature is useful in establishing that ovulation has occurred, but it should not be used to predict the onset of ovulation in a given cycle.

2. Another test used to assess ovulation is a midluteal phase serum progesterone concentration. A blood sample is usually obtained for progesterone 7 days after the estimated day of ovulation. A concentration greater than 3.0 ng/mL is consistent with ovulation, while a concentration greater than 10 ng/mL signifies adequate luteal phase support.

3. Alternatively, urine LH kits can be used to assess ovulation. Unlike the rise in BBT and serum progesterone concentrations, which are useful for retrospectively documenting ovulation, urinary LH kits can be used to predict ovulation. Ovulation usually occurs 24 to 36 hours after detecting the LH surge.

H. Tubal patency can be evaluated by hysterosalpingography (HSG) and/or by chromopertubation during laparoscopy.

Timing of the Infertility Evaluation	
Test	**Day**
Hysterosalpingogram	day 7-10
Postcoital Test	day 12-14
Serum Progesterone	day 21-23
Endometrial Biopsy	day 25-28

II. Differential diagnosis and treatment

A. The differential diagnosis of infertility includes ovarian (20%), pelvic (25%), cervical (10%), and male (35%) factors. In approximately 10% of cases no explanation is found. Optimal frequency of coitus is every other day around the time of ovulation; however, comparable pregnancy rates are achieved by 3-4 times weekly intercourse throughout the cycle.

B. Ovarian factor infertility

1. An ovarian factor is suggested by irregular cycles, abnormal BBT charts, midluteal phase serum progesterone levels less than 3 ng/mL, or luteal phase defect documented by endometrial biopsy. Ovulatory dysfunction may be intrinsic to the ovaries or caused by thyroid, adrenal, prolactin, or central nervous system disorders. Emotional stress, changes in weight, or excessive exercise should be sought because these disorders can result in ovulatory dysfunction. Luteal phase deficiency is most often the result of inadequate ovarian progesterone secretion.

2. **Clomiphene citrate (Clomid, CC)** is the most cost-effective treatment for the treatment of infertility related to anovulation or oligo ovulation. The usual starting dose of CC is 50 mg/day for 5 days, beginning on the second to sixth day after induced or spontaneous bleeding. Ovulation is expected between 7 and 10 days after the last dose of CC.

3. Ovulation on a specified dosage of CC should be confirmed with a midluteal phase serum progesterone assay, BBT rise, pelvic ultrasonography, or urinary ovulation-predictor kits. In the event ovulation does not occur with a specified dose of CC, the dose can be increased by 50 mg/day in a subsequent cycle. The maximum dose of CC should not exceed 250 mg/day. The addition of dexamethasone is advocated for women with elevated dehydroepiandrosterone sulfate levels who remain anovulatory despite high doses of CC. The incidence of multiple gestations with CC is 5% to 10%. Approximately 33% of patients will become pregnant within five cycles of treatment. Treatment with CC for more than six ovulatory cycles is not recommended because of low success rates.

4. **Human menopausal gonadotropins (hMG, Pergonal, Metrodin)** ovulation induction with is another option for the treatment of ovulatory dysfunction. Because of its expense and associated risk of multiple gestations, gonadotropin therapy should be reserved for patients who remain refractory to CC therapy. The pregnancy rate with gonadotropin therapy is 25% per cycle. This is most likely the result of recruitment of more follicles with gonadotropin therapy. The incidence of multiple gestations with gonadotropin therapy is 25% to 30%.

5. **Luteal phase deficiency** is treated with progesterone, usually prescribed as an intravaginal suppository at a dose of 25 mg twice a day until 8 to 10 weeks of gestation.

6. **Women with ovulatory dysfunction** secondary to ovarian failure or poor ovarian reserve should consider obtaining oocytes from a donor source.

C. Pelvic factor infertility

1. Pelvic factor infertility is caused by conditions that affect the fallopian tubes, peritoneum, or uterus. Tubal factor infertility is a common sequela of salpingitis. Appendicitis, ectopic pregnancy, endometriosis, and previous pelvic or abdominal surgery can also damage the fallopian tubes and cause adhesion formation.

2. Endometriosis is another condition involving the peritoneal cavity that is commonly associated with infertility. Uterine abnormalities are responsible for infertility in about 2% of cases. Examples of uterine abnormalities associated with infertility are congenital deformities of the uterus, leiomyomas, and intrauterine scarification or adhesions (Asherman's syndrome).

3. The mainstay of treatment of pelvic factor infertility relies on laparoscopy and hysteroscopy. In many instances, tubal reconstructive surgery, lysis of adhesions, and ablation and resection of endometriosis can be accomplished laparoscopically.

D. Cervical factor infertility

1. Cervical factor infertility is suggested when well-timed PCTs are consistently abnormal in the presence of a normal semen analysis. Cervical factor infertility results from inadequate mucus production by the cervical epithelium, poor mucus quality, or the presence of antisperm antibodies.

2. Patients with an abnormal PCT should be screened for an infectious etiology. The presence of immotile sperm or sperm shaking in place and not demonstrating forward motion is suggestive of immunologically related infertility. Sperm-cervical mucus and antisperm antibody testing are indicated when PCTs are repeatedly abnormal, despite normal-appearing cervical mucus and normal semen analysis.

E. Male factor infertility
includes conditions that affect sperm production, sperm maturation, and sperm delivery. Intrauterine insemination is frequently used to treat men with impaired semen parameters.

F. Unexplained Infertility

1. The term unexplained infertility should be used only after a thorough infertility investigation has failed to reveal an identifiable source and the duration of infertility is 24 months or more. History, physical examination, documentation of ovulation, endometrial biopsy, semen analyses, PCT, hysterosalpingogram, and laparoscopy should have been completed.

2. Because couples with unexplained infertility lack an identifiable causative factor of their infertility, empirical treatment with clomiphene therapy increases the spontaneous pregnancy rate to 6.8% per cycle compared with 2.8% in placebo-control cycles. For optimal results, gonadotropins should be used for ovulation induction. Intrauterine insemination, in vitro fertilization and gamete intrafallopian transfer (GIFT) are additional options.

References: See page 166.

Sexual Dysfunction

Almost two-thirds of the women may have had sexual difficulties at some time. Fifteen percent of women experience pain with intercourse, 18-48% experience difficulty becoming aroused, 46% note difficulty reaching orgasm, and 15-24% are not orgasmic.

I. **Clinical evaluation of sexual dysfunction.** Sexual difficulty can be caused by a lack of communication, insufficient stimulation, a lack of understanding of sexual response, lack of nurturing, physical discomfort, or fear of infection.

II. Treatment of sexual dysfunction
A. Lack of arousal
1. Difficulty becoming sexually aroused may occur if there is insufficient foreplay or if either partner is emotionally distracted. Arousal phase dysfunction may be manifest by insufficient vasocongestion.
2. Treatment consists of Sensate Focus exercises. In these exercises, the woman and her partner take turns caressing each other's body, except for the genital area. When caressing becomes pleasurable for both partners, they move on to manual genital stimulation, and then to further sexual activity.

B. Lack of orgasm
1. Lack of orgasm should be considered a problem if the patient or her partner perceives it as one. Ninety percent of women are able to experience orgasm.
2. **At-home methods of overcoming dysfunction**
   a. The patient should increase self-awareness by examining her body and genitals at home. The patient should identify sensitive areas that produce pleasurable feelings. The intensity and duration of psychologic stimulation may be increased by sexual fantasy.
   b. If, after completing the above steps, an orgasm has not been reached, the patient may find that the use of a vibrator on or around the clitoris is effective.
   c. Once masturbation has resulted in orgasm, the patient should masturbate with her partner present and demonstrate pleasurable stimulation techniques.
   d. Once high levels of arousal have been achieved, the couple may engage in intercourse. Manual stimulation of the clitoris during intercourse may be beneficial.

C. Dyspareunia
1. Dyspareunia consists of pain during intercourse. Organic disorders that may contribute to dyspareunia include hypoestrogenism, endometriosis, ovaries located in the cul-de-sac, fibroids, and pelvic infection.
2. Evaluation for dyspareunia should include careful assessment of the genital tract and an attempt to reproduce symptoms during bimanual examination.

D. Vaginismus
1. Vaginismus consists of spasm of the levator ani muscle, making penetration into the vagina painful. Some women may be unable to undergo pelvic examination.
2. **Treatment of vaginismus**
   a. **Vaginal dilators.** Plastic syringe covers or vaginal dilators are available in sets of 4 graduated sizes. The smallest dilator (the size of the fifth finger) is placed in the vagina by the woman. As each dilator is replaced with the next larger size without pain, muscle relaxation occurs.
   b. **Muscle awareness exercises**
      (1) The examiner places one finger inside the vaginal introitus, and the woman is instructed to contract the muscle that she uses to stop urine flow. The woman then inserts her own finger into the vagina and contracts. The process is continued at home.
      (2) Once a woman can identify the appropriate muscles, vaginal contractions can be done without placing a finger in the vagina.

E. Medications that interfere with sexual function. The most common of medications that interfere with sexual function are antihypertensive agents, anti-psychotics, and antidepressants.

Medications Associated With Sexual Dysfunction in Women		
Medication	**Decreased Li-bido**	**Delayed or No Orgasm**
Amphetamines and anorexic drugs		X
Cimetidine	X	
Diazepam		X
Fluoxetine		X
Imipramine		X
Propranolol	X	

References: See page 166.

Urinary Incontinence

Women between the ages of 20 to 80 year have an overall prevalence for urinary incontinence of 53.2 percent.

I. Types of Urinary Incontinence
   A. Stress Incontinence
      1. Stress incontinence is the involuntary loss of urine produced by coughing, laughing or exercising. The underlying abnormality is typically urethral hypermobility caused by a failure of the anatomic supports of the bladder neck. Loss of bladder neck support is often attributed to injury occurring during vaginal delivery.
      2. The lack of normal intrinsic pressure within the urethra--known as intrinsic urethral sphincter deficiency--is another factor leading to stress incontinence. Advanced age, inadequate estrogen levels, previous vaginal surgery and certain neurologic lesions are associated with poor urethral sphincter function.
   B. Overactive Bladder. Involuntary loss of urine preceded by a strong urge to void, whether or not the bladder is full, is a symptom of the condition commonly referred to as "urge incontinence." Other commonly used terms such as detrusor instability and detrusor hyperreflexia refer to involuntary detrusor contractions observed during urodynamic studies.
II. History and Physical Examination
   A. A preliminary diagnosis of urinary incontinence can be made on the basis of a history, physical examination and a few simple office and laboratory tests.
   B. The medical history should assess diabetes, stroke, lumbar disc disease, chronic lung disease, fecal impaction and cognitive impairment. The obstetric and gynecologic history should include gravity; parity; the number of vaginal, instrument-assisted and cesarean deliveries; the time interval between deliveries; previous hysterectomy and/or vaginal or bladder surgery; pelvic radiotherapy; trauma; and estrogen status.

Key Questions in Evaluating Patients for Urinary Incontinence

Do you leak urine when you cough, laugh, lift something or sneeze? How often?
Do you ever leak urine when you have a strong urge on the way to the bathroom? How often?
How frequently do you empty your bladder during the day?
How many times do you get up to urinate after going to sleep? Is it the urge to urinate that wakes you?
Do you ever leak urine during sex?
Do you wear pads that protect you from leaking urine? How often do you have to change them?
Do you ever find urine on your pads or clothes and were unaware of when the leakage occurred?
Does it hurt when you urinate?
Do you ever feel that you are unable to completely empty your bladder?

Drugs That Can Influence Bladder Function

Drug	Side effect
Antidepressants, antipsychotics, sedatives/hypnotics	Sedation, retention (overflow)
Diuretics	Frequency, urgency (OAB)
Caffeine	Frequency, urgency (OAB)
Anticholinergics	Retention (overflow)
Alcohol	Sedation, frequency (OAB)
Narcotics	Retention, constipation, sedation (OAB and overflow)
Alpha-adrenergic blockers	Decreased urethral tone (stress incontinence)
Alpha-adrenergic agonists	Increased urethral tone, retention (overflow)
Beta-adrenergic agonists	Inhibited detrusor function, retention (overflow)

C. Because fecal impaction has been linked to urinary incontinence, a history that includes frequency of bowel movements, length of time to evacuate and whether the patient must splint her vagina or perineum during defecation should be obtained. Patients should be questioned about fecal incontinence.

D. A complete list of all prescription and nonprescription drugs should be obtained. When appropriate, discontinuation of these medications associated with incontinence or substitution of appropriate alternative medications will often cure or significantly improve urinary incontinence.

E. **Physical Examination**
   1. Immediately before the physical examination, the patient should void as normally and completely as possible. The voided volume should be recorded. A post-void residual volume can then be determined within 10 minutes by catheterization or ultrasound examination. Post-void residual volumes more than 100 mL are considered abnormal.
   2. A clean urine sample can be sent for culture and urinalysis.
   3. Determining post-void residual volume and urinalysis allows screening

for overflow incontinence, chronic urinary tract infections, hematuria, diabetes, kidney disease and metabolic abnormalities.

4. The abdominal examination should rule out diastasis recti, masses, ascites and organomegaly. Pulmonary and cardiovascular assessment may be indicated to assess control of cough or the need for medications such as diuretics.

5. The lumbosacral nerve roots should be assessed by checking deep tendon reflexes, lower extremity strength, sharp/dull sensation and the bulbocavernosus and clitoral sacral reflexes.

6. The pelvic examination should include an evaluation for inflammation, infection and atrophy. Signs of inadequate estrogen levels are thinning and paleness of the vaginal epithelium, loss of rugae, disappearance of the labia minora and presence of a urethral caruncle.

7. A urethral diverticula is usually identified as a distal bulge under the urethra. Gentle massage of the area will frequently produce a purulent discharge from the urethral meatus.

8. Testing for stress incontinence is performed by asking the patient to cough vigorously while the examiner watches for leakage of urine.

9. While performing the bimanual examination, levator ani muscle function can be evaluated by asking the patient to tighten her "vaginal muscles" and hold the contraction as long as possible. It is normal for a woman to be able to hold such a contraction for five to 10 seconds. The bimanual examination should also include a rectal examination to assess anal sphincter tone, fecal impaction, occult blood, or rectal lesions.

III. **Treatment of urinary incontinence**
   A. Rehabilitation of the pelvic floor muscles is the common goal of treatments through the use of pelvic muscle exercises (Kegel's exercises), weighted vaginal cones and pelvic floor electrical stimulation.
   B. A set of specially designed vaginal weights can be used as mechanical biofeedback to augment pelvic muscle exercises. The weights are held inside the vagina by contracting the pelvic muscles for 15 minutes at a time.
   C. Pelvic floor electrical stimulation with a vaginal or anal probe produces a contraction of the levator ani muscle. Cure or improvement in 48 percent of treated patients, compared with 13 percent of control subjects.
   D. Occlusive devices, such as pessaries, can mimic the effects of a retropubic urethropexy. A properly fitted pessary prevents urine loss during vigorous coughing in the standing position with a full bladder.
   E. Medications such as estrogens and alpha-adrenergic drugs may also be effective in treating women with stress incontinence. Stress incontinence may be treated with localized estrogen replacement therapy (ERT). Localized ERT can be given in the form of estrogen cream or an estradiol-impregnated vaginal ring (Estring).

Medications Used to Treat Urinary Incontinence	
Drug	**Dosage**
Stress Incontinence	
Pseudoephedrine (Sudafed)	15 to 30 mg, three times daily
Vaginal estrogen ring (Estring)	Insert into vagina every three months.
Vaginal estrogen cream	0.5 g, apply in vagina every night

Drug	Dosage
Overactive bladder	
Oxybutynin ER (Ditropan XL)	5 to 15 mg, every morning
Tolterodine LA (Detrol LA)	2-4 mg qd
Generic oxybutynin	2.5 to 10 mg, two to four times daily
Tolterodine (Detrol)	1 to 2 mg, two times daily
Imipramine (Tofranil)	10 to 75 mg, every night
Dicyclomine (Bentyl)	10 to 20 mg, four times daily
Hyoscyamine (Cystospaz)	0.375 mg, two times daily

F. Alpha-adrenergic drugs such as pseudoephedrine improve stress incontinence by increase resting urethral tone. These drugs cause subjective improvement in 20 to 60 percent of patients.

G. Surgery to correct genuine stress incontinence is a viable option for most patients. Retropubic urethropexies (ie, Burch laparoscopic and Marshall-Marchetti-Krantz [MMK] procedures) and suburethral slings have long-term success rates consistently reported in the 80 to 96 percent range.

H. Another minimally invasive procedure for the treatment of stress incontinence caused by intrinsic sphincter deficiency is periurethral injection.

I. **Overactive bladder**

1. Behavioral therapy, in the form of bladder retraining and biofeedback, seeks to reestablish cortical control of the bladder by having the patient ignore urgency and void only in response to cortical signals during waking hours.

2. Pharmacologic agents may be given empirically to women with symptoms of overactive bladder. Tolterodine (Detrol) and extended-release oxybutynin chloride (Ditropan XL) have largely replaced generic oxybutynin as a first-line treatment option for overactive bladder because of favorable side effect profiles.

3. ERT is also an effective treatment for women with overactive bladder. Even in patients taking systemic estrogen, localized ERT (ie, estradiol-impregnated vaginal ring) may increase inadequate estrogen levels and decrease the symptoms associated with overactive bladder.

4. Pelvic floor electrical stimulation is also effective in treating women with overactive bladder. Pelvic floor electrical stimulation results in a 50 percent cure rate of detrusor instability.

5. Neuromodulation of the sacral nerve roots through electrodes implanted in the sacral foramina is a promising new surgical treatment that has been found to be effective in the treatment of urge incontinence.

6. The FDA has recently approved extracorporeal magnetic innervation, a noninvasive procedure for the treatment of incontinence caused by pelvic floor weakness. Extracorporeal magnetic innervation may have a place in the treatment of women with both stress and urge incontinence.

References: See page 166.

Urinary Tract Infection

Urinary tract infections (UTIs) are a leading cause of morbidity in persons of all ages. Sexually active young women, elderly persons and those undergoing genitourinary instrumentation or catheterization are at risk.

I. **Acute uncomplicated cystitis in young women**
   A. Sexually active young women are most at risk for UTIs.
   B. Approximately 90 percent of uncomplicated cystitis episodes are caused by Escherichia coli, 10 to 20 percent are caused by coagulase-negative Staphylococcus saprophyticus and 5 percent or less are caused by other Enterobacteriaceae organisms or enterococci. Up to one-third of uropathogens are resistant to ampicillin and, but the majority are susceptible to trimethoprim-sulfamethoxazole (85 to 95 percent) and fluoroquinolones (95 percent).
   C. Patients should be evaluated for pyuria by urinalysis (wet mount examination of spun urine) or a dipstick test for leukocyte esterase.

Urinary Tract Infections in Adults			
Category	Diagnostic criteria	First-line therapy	Comments
Acute uncomplicated cystitis	Urinalysis for pyuria and hematuria (culture not required)	TMP-SMX DS (Bactrim, Septra) Trimethoprim (Proloprim) Ciprofloxacin (Cipro) Ofloxacin (Floxin)	Three-day course is best Quinolones may be used in areas of TMP-SMX resistance or in patients who cannot tolerate TMP-SMX
Recurrent cystitis in young women	Symptoms and a urine culture with a bacterial count of more than 100 CFU per mL of urine	If the patient has more than three cystitis episodes per year, treat prophylactically with postcoital, patient-directed or continuous daily therapy	Repeat therapy for seven to 10 days based on culture results and then use prophylactic therapy
Acute cystitis in young men	Urine culture with a bacterial count of 1,000 to 10,000 CFU per mL of urine	Same as for acute uncomplicated cystitis	Treat for seven to 10 days
Acute uncomplicated pyelonephritis	Urine culture with a bacterial count of 100,000 CFU per mL of urine	If gram-negative organism, oral fluoroquinolone If gram-positive organism, amoxicillin If parenteral administration is required, ceftriaxone (Rocephin) or a fluoroquinolone If Enterococcus species, add oral or IV amoxicillin	Switch from IV to oral administration when the patient is able to take medication by mouth; complete a 14-day course

Category	Diagnostic criteria	First-line therapy	Comments
Complicated urinary tract infection	Urine culture with a bacterial count of more than 10,000 CFU per mL of urine	If gram-negative organism, oral fluoroquinolone If Enterococcus species, ampicillin or amoxicillin with or without gentamicin (Garamycin)	Treat for 10 to 14 days
Catheter-associated urinary tract infection	Symptoms and a urine culture with a bacterial count of more than 100 CFU per mL of urine	If gram-negative organism, a fluoroquinolone If gram-positive organism, ampicillin or amoxicillin plus gentamicin	Remove catheter if possible, and treat for seven to 10 days For patients with long-term catheters and symptoms, treat for five to seven days

Antibiotic Therapy for Urinary Tract Infections

Diagnostic group	Duration of therapy	Empiric options
Acute uncomplicated urinary tract infections in women	Three days	Trimethoprim-sulfamethoxazole (Bactrim DS), one double-strength tablet PO twice daily Trimethoprim (Proloprim), 100 mg PO twice daily Norfloxacin (Noroxin), 400 mg twice daily Ciprofloxacin (Cipro), 250 mg twice daily Lomefloxacin (Maxaquin), 400 mg per day Ofloxacin (Floxin), 200 mg twice daily Enoxacin (Penetrex), 200 mg twice daily Sparfloxacin (Zagam), 400 mg as initial dose, then 200 mg per day Levofloxacin (Levaquin), 250 mg per day Nitrofurantoin (Macrodantin), 100 mg four times daily Cefpodoxime (Vantin), 100 mg twice daily Cefixime (Suprax), 400 mg per day Amoxicillin-clavulanate (Augmentin), 500 mg twice daily
Acute uncomplicated pyelonephritis	14 days	Trimethoprim-sulfamethoxazole DS, one double-strength tablet PO twice daily Ciprofloxacin (Cipro), 500 mg twice daily Levofloxacin (Maxiquin), 250 mg per day Enoxacin (Penetrex), 400 mg twice daily Sparfloxacin (Zagam) 400 mg initial dose, then 200 mg per day 104.50 Ofloxacin (Floxin), 400 mg twice daily Cefpodoxime (Vantin), 200 mg twice daily Cefixime (Suprax), 400 mg per day

	Up to 3 days	Trimethoprim-sulfamethoxazole (Bactrim) 160/800 IV twice daily Ceftriaxone (Rocephin), 1 g IV per day Ciprofloxacin (Cipro), 400 mg twice daily Ofloxacin (Floxin), 400 mg twice daily Levofloxacin (Penetrex), 250 mg per day Aztreonam (Azactam), 1 g three times daily Gentamicin (Garamycin), 3 mg per kg per day in 3 divided doses every 8 hours
Complicated urinary tract infections	14 days	Fluoroquinolones PO
	Up to 3 days	Ampicillin, 1 g IV every six hours, and gentamicin, 3 mg per kg per day
Urinary tract infections in young men	Seven days	Trimethoprim-sulfamethoxazole, one double-strength tablet PO twice daily Fluoroquinolones

D. Treatment of acute uncomplicated cystitis in young women
   1. Three-day regimens appear to offer the optimal combination of convenience, low cost and an efficacy comparable to that of seven-day or longer regimens.
   2. Trimethoprim-sulfamethoxazole is the most cost-effective treatment. Three-day regimens of ciprofloxacin (Cipro), 250 mg twice daily, and ofloxacin (Floxin), 200 mg twice daily, produce better cure rates with less toxicity.
   3. Quinolones that are useful in treating complicated and uncomplicated cystitis include ciprofloxacin, norfloxacin, ofloxacin, enoxacin (Penetrex), lomefloxacin (Maxaquin), sparfloxacin (Zagam) and levofloxacin (Levaquin).
   4. Trimethoprim-sulfamethoxazole remains the antibiotic of choice in the treatment of uncomplicated UTIs in young women. Fluoroquinolones are recommended for patients who cannot tolerate sulfonamides or trimethoprim or who have a high frequency of antibiotic resistance. Three days is the optimal duration of treatment for uncomplicated cystitis. A seven-day course should be considered in pregnant women, diabetic women and women who have had symptoms for more than one week.

II. Recurrent cystitis in young women
   A. Up to 20 percent of young women with acute cystitis develop recurrent UTIs. The causative organism should be identified by urine culture.
   B. Women who have more than three UTI recurrences within one year can be managed using one of three preventive strategies.
      1. Acute self-treatment with a three-day course of standard therapy.
      2. Postcoital prophylaxis with one-half of a trimethoprim-sulfamethoxazole double-strength tablet (40/200 mg).
      3. Continuous daily prophylaxis for six months with trimethoprim-sulfamethoxazole, one-half tablet per day (40/200 mg); nitrofurantoin, 50 to 100 mg per day; norfloxacin (Noroxin), 200 mg per day; cephalexin (Keflex), 250 mg per day; or trimethoprim (Proloprim), 100 mg per day.

III. Complicated UTI
   A. A complicated UTI is one that occurs because of enlargement of the prostate gland, blockages, or the presence of resistant bacteria.
   B. Accurate urine culture and susceptibility are necessary. Treatment consists of an oral fluoroquinolone. In patients who require hospitalization, parenteral administration of ceftazidime (Fortaz) or cefoperazone (Cefobid), cefepime (Maxipime), aztreonam (Azactam), imipenem-cilastatin (Primaxin) or the combination of an antipseudomonal penicillin (ticarcillin [Ticar], mezlocillin [Mezlin], piperacillin [Pipracil]) with an aminoglycoside.

    C. Enterococci are frequently encountered uropathogens in complicated UTIs. In areas in which vancomycin-resistant Enterococcus faecium is prevalent, quinupristin-dalfopristin (Synercid) may be useful.

    D. Patients with complicated UTIs require at least a 10- to 14-day course of therapy. Follow-up urine cultures should be performed within 10 to 14 days after treatment.

IV. Uncomplicated pyelonephritis

    A. Women with acute uncomplicated pyelonephritis may present with a mild cystitis-like illness and flank pain; fever, chills, nausea, vomiting, leukocytosis and abdominal pain; or a serious gram-negative bacteremia. Uncomplicated pyelonephritis is usually caused by E. coli.

    B. The diagnosis should be confirmed by urinalysis and by urine culture. Urine cultures demonstrate more than 100,000 CFU per mL of urine in 80 percent of women with pyelonephritis. Blood cultures are positive in up to 20 percent of women who have this infection.

    C. Empiric therapy using an oral fluoroquinolone is recommended in women with mild to moderate symptoms. Patients who are too ill to take oral antibiotics should initially be treated with a parenterally third-generation cephalosporin, aztreonam, a broad-spectrum penicillin, a quinolone or an aminoglycoside.

    D. The total duration of therapy is usually 14 days. Patients with persistent symptoms after three days of antimicrobial therapy should be evaluated by renal ultrasonography for evidence of urinary obstruction or abscess.

References: See page 166.

Pubic Infections

I. Molluscum contagiosum

    A. This disease is produced by a virus of the pox virus family and is spread by sexual or close personal contact. Lesions are usually asymptomatic and multiple, with a central umbilication. Lesions can be spread by autoinoculation and last from 6 months to many years.

    B. Diagnosis. The characteristic appearance is adequate for diagnosis, but biopsy may be used to confirm the diagnosis.

    C. Treatment. Lesions are removed by sharp dermal curette, liquid nitrogen cryosurgery, or electrodesiccation.

II. Pediculosis pubis (crabs)

    A. Phthirus pubis is a blood sucking louse that is unable to survive more than 24 hours off the body. It is often transmitted sexually and is principally found on the pubic hairs. Diagnosis is confirmed by locating nits or adult lice on the hair shafts.

    B. Treatment

        1. Permethrin cream (Elimite), 5% is the most effective treatment; it is applied for 10 minutes and washed off.

        2. Kwell shampoo, lathered for at least 4 minutes, can also be used, but it is contraindicated in pregnancy or lactation.

        3. All contaminated clothing and linen should be laundered.

III. Pubic scabies

    A. This highly contagious infestation is caused by the Sarcoptes scabiei (0.2-0.4 mm in length). The infestation is transmitted by intimate contact or by contact with infested clothing. The female mite burrows into the skin, and after 1 month, severe pruritus develops. A multiform eruption may develop, characterized by papules, vesicles, pustules, urticarial wheals, and secondary infections on the hands, wrists, elbows, belt line, buttocks, genitalia, and outer feet.

    B. Diagnosis is confirmed by visualization of burrows and observation of parasites, eggs, larvae, or red fecal compactions under microscopy.

    C. Treatment. Permethrin 5% cream (Elimite) is massaged in from the neck down and remove by washing after 8 hours.

References: See page 166.

Sexually Transmissible Infections

Approximately 12 million patients are diagnosed with a sexually transmissible infection (STI) annually in the United States. Sequella of STIs include infertility, chronic pelvic pain, ectopic pregnancy, and other adverse pregnancy outcomes.

Diagnosis and Treatment of Bacterial Sexually Transmissible Infections

Organism	Diagnostic Methods	Recommended Treatment	Alternative
Chlamydia trachomatis	Direct fluorescent antibody, enzyme immunoassay, DNA probe, cell culture, DNA amplification	Doxycycline 100 mg PO 2 times a day for 7 days or Azithromycin (Zithromax) 1 g PO	Ofloxacin (Floxin) 300 mg PO 2 times a day for 7 days
Neisseria gonorrhoeae	Culture DNA probe	Ceftriaxone (Rocephin) 125 mg IM or Cefixime 400 mg PO or Ciprofloxacin (Cipro) 500 mg PO or Ofloxacin (Floxin) 400 mg PO plus Doxycycline 100 mg 2 times a day for 7 days or azithromycin 1 g PO	Levofloxacin (Levaquin) 250 mg PO once Spectinomycin 2 g IM once
Treponema pallidum	Clinical appearance Dark-field microscopy Nontreponemal test: rapid plasma reagin, VDRL Treponemal test: MHA-TP, FTA-ABS	Primary and secondary syphilis and early latent syphilis (<1 year duration): benzathine penicillin G 2.4 million units IM in a single dose.	Penicillin allergy in patients with primary, secondary, or early latent syphilis (<1 year of duration): doxycycline 100 mg PO 2 times a day for 2 weeks.

Diagnosis and Treatment of Viral Sexually Transmissible Infections

Organism	Diagnostic Methods	Recommended Treatment Regimens
Herpes simplex virus	Clinical appearance Cell culture confirmation	First episode: Acyclovir (Zovirax) 400 mg PO 5 times a day for 7-10 days, or famciclovir (Famvir) 250 mg PO 3 times a day for 7-10 days, or valacyclovir (Valtrex) 1 g PO 2 times a day for 7-10 days. Recurrent episodes: acyclovir 400 mg PO 3 times a day for 5 days, or 800 mg PO 2 times a day for 5 days or famciclovir 125 mg PO 2 times a day for 5 days, or valacyclovir 500 mg PO 2 times a day for 5 days Daily suppressive therapy: acyclovir 400 mg PO 2 times a day, or famciclovir 250 mg PO 2 times a day, or valacyclovir 250 mg PO 2 times a day, 500 mg PO 1 time a day, or 1000 mg PO 1 time a day

Organism	Diagnostic Methods	Recommended Treatment Regimens
Human papilloma virus	Clinical appearance of condyloma papules Cytology	External warts: Patient may apply podofilox 0.5% solution or gel 2 times a day for 3 days, followed by 4 days of no therapy, for a total of up to 4 cycles, or imiquimod 5% cream at bedtime 3 times a week for up to 16 weeks. Cryotherapy with liquid nitrogen or cryoprobe, repeat every 1-2 weeks; or podophyllin, repeat weekly; or TCA 80-90%, repeat weekly; or surgical removal. Vaginal warts: cryotherapy with liquid nitrogen, or TCA 80-90%, or podophyllin 10-25%
Human immunodeficiency virus	Enzyme immunoassay Western blot (for confirmation) Polymerase chain reaction	Antiretroviral agents

Treatment of Pelvic Inflammatory Disease		
Regimen	Inpatient	Outpatient
A	Cefotetan (Cefotan) 2 g IV q12h; or cefoxitin (Mefoxin) 2 g IV q6h plus doxycycline 100 mg IV or PO q12h.	Ofloxacin (Floxin) 400 mg PO bid for 14 days plus metronidazole 500 mg PO bid for 14 days.
B	Clindamycin 900 mg IV q8h plus gentamicin loading dose IV or IM (2 mg/kg of body weight), followed by a maintenance dose (1.5 mg/kg) q8h.	Ceftriaxone (Rocephin) 250 mg IM once; or cefoxitin 2 g IM plus probenecid 1 g PO; or other parenteral third-generation cephalosporin (eg, ceftizoxime, cefotaxime) plus doxycycline 100 mg PO bid for 14 days.

I. **Chlamydia Trachomatis**
   A. Chlamydia trachomatis is the most prevalent STI in the United States. Chlamydial infections are most common in women age 15-19 years.
   B. Routine screening of asymptomatic, sexually active adolescent females undergoing pelvic examination is recommended. Annual screening should be done for women age 20-24 years who are either inconsistent users of barrier contraceptives or who acquired a new sex partner or had more than one sexual partner in the past 3 months.
II. **Gonorrhea.** Gonorrhea has an incidence of 800,000 cases annually. Routine screening for gonorrhea is recommended among women at high risk of infection, including prostitutes, women with a history of repeated episodes of gonorrhea, women under age 25 years with two or more sex partners in the past year, and women with mucopurulent cervicitis.
III. **Syphilis**
   A. Syphilis has an incidence of 100,000 cases annually. The rates are highest in the South, among African Americans, and among those in the 20- to 24-year-old age group.
   B. Prostitutes, persons with other STIs, and sexual contacts of persons with active syphilis should be screened.
IV. **Herpes simplex virus and human papillomavirus**
   A. An estimated 200,000-500,000 new cases of herpes simplex occur annually in the United States. New infections are most common in adolescents and young adults.

B. Human papillomavirus affects about 30% of young, sexually active individuals.

References: See page 166.

Pelvic Inflammatory Disease

Pelvic inflammatory disease (PID) is an acute infection of the upper genital tract in women, involving any or all of the uterus, oviducts, and ovaries. PID is a community-acquired infection initiated by a sexually transmitted agent. Pelvic inflammatory disease accounts for approximately 2.5 million outpatient visits and 200,000 hospitalizations annually.

I. **Clinical evaluation**
   A. Lower abdominal pain is the cardinal presenting symptom in women with PID, although the character of the pain may be quite subtle. The onset of pain during or shortly after menses is particularly suggestive. The abdominal pain is usually bilateral and rarely of more than two weeks' duration.
   B. Abnormal uterine bleeding occurs in one-third or more of patients with PID. New vaginal discharge, urethritis, proctitis, fever, and chills can be associated signs.
   C. Risk factors for PID:
      1. Age less than 35 years
      2. Nonbarrier contraception
      3. New, multiple, or symptomatic sexual partners
      4. Previous episode of PID
      5. Oral contraception
      6. African-American ethnicity
II. **Physical examination**
   A. Only one-half of patients with PID have fever. Abdominal examination reveals diffuse tenderness greatest in the lower quadrants, which may or may not be symmetrical. Rebound tenderness and decreased bowel sounds are common. Tenderness in the right upper quadrant does not exclude PID, because approximately 10 percent of these patients have perihepatitis (Fitz-Hugh Curtis syndrome).
   B. Purulent endocervical discharge and/or acute cervical motion and adnexal tenderness by bimanual examination is strongly suggestive of PID. Rectovaginal examination should reveal the uterine adnexal tenderness.
III. **Diagnosis**
   A. Diagnostic criteria and guidelines. The index of suspicion for the clinical diagnosis of PID should be high, especially in adolescent women.
   B. The CDC has recommended minimum criteria required for empiric treatment of PID. These major determinants include lower abdominal tenderness, adnexal tenderness, and cervical motion tenderness. Minor determinants (ie, signs that may increase the suspicion of PID) include:
      1. Fever (oral temperature >101°F; >38.3°C)
      2. Vaginal discharge
      3. Documented STD
      4. Erythrocyte sedimentation rate (ESR)
      5. C-reactive protein
      6. Systemic signs
      7. Dyspareunia
   C. Empiric treatment for pelvic inflammatory disease is recommended when:
      1. The examination suggests PID
      2. Demographics (risk factors) are consistent with PID

3. Pregnancy test is negative

Laboratory Evaluation for Pelvic Inflammatory Disease

- Pregnancy test
- Microscopic exam of vaginal discharge in saline
- Complete blood counts
- Tests for chlamydia and gonococcus
- Urinalysis
- Fecal occult blood test
- C-reactive protein(optional)

IV. Diagnostic testing

    A. Laboratory testing for patients suspected of having PID always begins with a pregnancy test to rule out ectopic pregnancy and complications of an intrauterine pregnancy. A urinalysis and a stool for occult blood should be obtained because abnormalities in either reduce the probability of PID. Blood counts have limited value. Fewer than one-half of PID patients exhibit leukocytosis.

    B. Gram stain and microscopic examination of vaginal discharge may provide useful information. If a cervical Gram stain is positive for Gram-negative intracellular diplococci, the probability of PID greatly increases; if negative, it is of little use.

    C. Increased white blood cells (WBC) in vaginal fluid may be the most sensitive single laboratory test for PID (78 percent for ≥3 WBC per high power field). However, the specificity is only 39 percent.

    D. Recommended laboratory tests:

        1. Pregnancy test

        2. Microscopic exam of vaginal discharge in saline

        3. Complete blood counts

        4. Tests for chlamydia and gonococcus

        5. Urinalysis

        6. Fecal occult blood test

        7. C-reactive protein(optional)

    E. Ultrasound imaging is reserved for acutely ill patients with PID in whom a pelvic abscess is a consideration.

V. Recommendations

    A. Health care providers should maintain a low threshold for the diagnosis of PID, and sexually active young women with lower abdominal, adnexal, and cervical motion tenderness should receive empiric treatment. The specificity of these clinical criteria can be enhanced by the presence of fever, abnormal cervical/vaginal discharge, elevated ESR and/or serum C-reactive protein, and the demonstration of cervical gonorrhea or chlamydia infection.

    B. If clinical findings (epidemiologic, symptomatic, and physical examination) suggest PID empiric treatment should be initiated.

Differential Diagnosis of Pelvic Inflammatory Disease

Appendicitis	Irritable bowel syndrome
Ectopic pregnancy	Somatization
Hemorrhagic ovarian cyst	Gastroenteritis
Ovarian torsion	Cholecystitis
Endometriosis	Nephrolithiasis
Urinary tract Infection	

VI. Treatment of pelvic inflammatory disease

    A. The two most important initiators of PID, Neisseria gonorrhoeae and Chlamydia trachomatis, must be treated, but coverage should also be provided for groups A and B streptococci, Gram negative enteric bacilli

(Escherichia coli, Klebsiella spp., and Proteus spp.), and anaerobes.

B. Outpatient therapy
1. For outpatient therapy, the CDC recommends either oral ofloxacin (Floxin, 400 mg twice daily) or levofloxacin (Levaquin, 500 mg once daily) with or without metronidazole (Flagyl, 500 mg twice daily) for 14 days. An alternative is an initial single dose of ceftriaxone (Rocephin, 250 mg IM), cefoxitin (Mefoxin, 2 g IM plus probenecid 1 g orally), or another parenteral third-generation cephalosporin, followed by doxycycline (100 mg orally twice daily) with or without metronidazole for 14 days. Quinolones are not recommended to treat gonorrhea acquired in California or Hawaii. If the patient may have acquired the disease in Asia, Hawaii, or California, cefixime or ceftriaxone should be used.
2. Another alternative is azithromycin (Zithromax, 1 g PO for Chlamydia coverage) and amoxicillin-clavulanate (Amoxicillin, 875 mg PO) once by directly observed therapy, followed by amoxicillin-clavulanate (Amoxicillin, 875 mg PO BID) for 7 to 10 days.

C. Inpatient therapy
1. For inpatient treatment, the CDC suggests either of the following regimens:
   a. **Cefotetan (Cefotan)**, 2 g IV Q12h, or cefoxitin (Mefoxin, 2 g IV Q6h) plus doxycycline (100 mg IV or PO Q12h)
   b. **Clindamycin (Cleocin)**, 900 mg IV Q8h, plus gentamicin (1-1.5 mg/kg IV q8h)
2. **Alternative regimens:**
   a. **Ofloxacin (Floxin)**, 400 mg IV Q12h or levofloxacin (Levaquin, 500 mg IV QD) with or without metronidazole (Flagyl, 500 mg IV Q8h). Quinolones are not recommended to treat gonorrhea acquired in California or Hawaii. If the patient may have acquired the disease in Asia, Hawaii, or California, cefixime or ceftriaxone should be used.
   b. **Ampicillin-sulbactam (Unasyn)**, 3 g IV Q6h plus doxycycline (100 mg IV or PO Q12h)
3. Parenteral administration of antibiotics should be continued for 24 hours after clinical response, followed by doxycycline (100 mg PO BID) or clindamycin (Cleocin, 450 mg PO QID) for a total of 14 days.
4. The following two regimens may also be used:
   a. **Levofloxacin (Levaquin)**, 500 mg IV Q24h, plus metronidazole (Flagyl, 500 mg IV Q8h). With this regimen, azithromycin (Zithromax, 1 g PO once) should be given as soon as the patient is tolerating oral intake. Parenteral therapy is continued until the pelvic tenderness on bimanual examination is mild or absent.

D. Annual screening is recommended for all sexually active women under age 25 and for women over 25 if they have new or multiple sexual partners. A retest for chlamydia should be completed in 3 to 4 months after chlamydia treatment because of high rates of reinfection.

E. Additional evaluation:
1. Serology for the human immunodeficiency virus (HIV)
2. Papanicolaou smear
3. Hepatitis B surface antigen determination and initiation of the vaccine series for patients who are antigen negative and unvaccinated
4. Hepatitis C virus serology
5. Serologic tests for syphilis

References: See page 166.

Vaginitis

Vaginitis is the most common gynecologic problem encountered by primary care physicians. It may result from bacterial infections, fungal infection, protozoan infection, contact dermatitis, atrophic vaginitis, or allergic reaction.

I. **Clinical evaluation of vaginal symptoms**
   A. The type and extent of symptoms, such as itching, discharge, odor, or pelvic pain should be determined. A change in sexual partners or sexual activity, changes in contraception method, medications (antibiotics), and history of prior genital infections should be sought.
   B. **Physical examination**
      1. Evaluation of the vagina should include close inspection of the external genitalia for excoriations, ulcerations, blisters, papillary structures, erythema, edema, mucosal thinning, or mucosal pallor.
      2. The color, texture, and odor of vaginal or cervical discharge should be noted.
   C. **Vaginal fluid pH** can be determined by immersing pH paper in the vaginal discharge. A pH level greater than 4.5 indicates the presence of bacterial vaginosis or Trichomonas vaginalis.
   D. **Saline wet mount**
      1. One swab should be used to obtain a sample from the posterior vaginal fornix, obtaining a "clump" of discharge. Place the sample on a slide, add one drop of normal saline, and apply a coverslip.
      2. Coccoid bacteria and clue cells (bacteria-coated, stippled, epithelial cells) are characteristic of bacterial vaginosis.
      3. Trichomoniasis is confirmed by identification of trichomonads – mobile, oval flagellates. White blood cells are prevalent.
   E. **Potassium hydroxide (KOH) preparation**
      1. Place a second sample on a slide, apply one drop of 10% potassium hydroxide (KOH) and a coverslip. A pungent, fishy odor upon addition of KOH – a positive whiff test – strongly indicates bacterial vaginosis.
      2. The KOH prep may reveal Candida in the form of thread-like hyphae and budding yeast.
   F. **Screening for STDs.** Testing for gonorrhea and chlamydial infection should be completed for women with a new sexual partner, purulent cervical discharge, or cervical motion tenderness.

II. **Differential diagnosis**
   A. The most common cause of vaginitis is bacterial vaginosis, followed by Candida albicans. The prevalence of trichomoniasis has declined in recent years.
   B. Common nonvaginal etiologies include contact dermatitis from spermicidal creams, latex in condoms, or douching. Any STD can produce vaginal discharge.

Clinical Manifestations of Vaginitis	
Candidal Vaginitis	Nonmalodorous, thick, white, "cottage cheese-like" discharge that adheres to vaginal walls Hyphal forms or budding yeast cells on wet-mount Pruritus Normal pH (<4.5)
Bacterial Vaginosis	Thin, dark or dull grey, homogeneous, malodorous discharge that adheres to the vaginal walls Elevated pH level (>4.5) Positive KOH (whiff test) Clue cells on wet-mount microscopic evaluation
Trichomonas Vaginalis	Copious, yellow-gray or green, homogeneous or frothy, malodorous discharge Elevated pH level (>4.5) Mobile, flagellated organisms and leukocytes on wet-mount microscopic evaluation Vulvovaginal irritation, dysuria
Atrophic Vaginitis	Vaginal dryness or burning

III. Yeast vaginitis

A. Half of all women have had at least one episode of yeast vaginitis. Candida albicans accounts for 80% of yeast infections. The remaining 20% are caused by Candida glabrata or Candida tropicalis. Pregnancy, oral contraceptives, antibiotics, diabetes and HIV infection are contributing factors.

B. **Diagnosis**
1. Typical symptoms are pruritus, thick vaginal discharge, and genital irritation. Discharge is odorless and cottage cheese-like. Women may complain of dysuria.
2. Physical examination may reveal vulvar erythema and fissuring.
3. Laboratory evaluation of vaginal fluid reveals a pH of less than 4.5 and the presence of hyphae on 10% potassium hydroxide (KOH) wet mount. Elevations in pH also occur in the presence of semen or blood.
4. Microscopy will reveal hyphae. The sensitivity of the KOH wet mount is only 50% to 70%. Therefore, treatment should be instituted even when hyphae are absent but the clinical impression is otherwise consistent.
5. Culture should be considered if the diagnosis is in doubt or in recurrent cases. Dermatophyte test medium is sensitive yeast.

C. **Treatment**
1. Uncomplicated vaginitis. These episodes can be treated with any nonprescription short-course (up to 7-day) preparation, since all are equally effective.

Treatment regimens for yeast vaginitis*

1-day regimens
Clotrimazole vaginal tablets (Mycelex G), 500 mg hs**
Fluconazole tablets (Diflucan), 150 mg PO
Itraconazole capsules (Sporanox), 200 mg PO bid
Tioconazole 6.5% vaginal ointment (Vagistat-1), 4.6 g hs** [5 g]

3-day regimens
Butoconazole nitrate 2% vaginal cream (Femstat 3), 5 g hs [28 g]
Clotrimazole vaginal inserts (Gyne-Lotrimin 3), 200 mg hs**
Miconazole vaginal suppositories (Monistat 3), 200 mg hs**
Terconazole 0.8% vaginal cream (Terazol 3), 5 g hs
Terconazole vaginal suppositories (Terazol 3), 80 mg hs
Itraconazole capsules (Sporanox), 200 mg PO qd (4)

5-day regimen
Ketoconazole tablets (Nizoral), 400 mg PO bid (4)

7-day regimens
Clotrimazole 1% cream (Gyne-Lotrimin, Mycelex-7, Sweet'n Fresh Clotrimazole-7), 5 g hs**
Clotrimazole vaginal tablets (Gyne-Lotrimin, Mycelex-7, Sweet'n Fresh Clotrimazole-7), 100 mg hs**
Miconazole 2% vaginal cream (Femizol-M, Monistat 7), 5 g hs**
Miconazole vaginal suppositories (Monistat 7), 100 mg hs**
Terconazole 0.4% vaginal cream (Terazol 7), 5 g hs

14-day regimens
Nystatin vaginal tablets (Mycostatin), 100,000 U hs
Boric acid No. 0 gelatin vaginal suppositories, 600 mg bid (2)

*Suppositories can be used if inflammation is predominantly vaginal; creams if vulvar; a combination if both. Cream-suppository combination packs available: clotrimazole (Gyne-Lotrimin, Mycelex); miconazole (Monistat, M-Zole). If diagnosis is in doubt, consider oral therapy to avoid amelioration of symptoms with use of creams. Use 1-day or 3-day regimen if compliance is an issue. Miconazole nitrate may be used during pregnancy.

**Nonprescription formulation. If nonprescription therapies fail, use terconazole 0.4% cream or 80-mg suppositories at bedtime for 7 days.

---

   2. Complicated infections are more severe and cure is more difficult. With use of nonprescription preparations, the treatment course should be longer (10 to 14 days). Since Candida species other than albicans may be more likely in complicated infections, treatment with terconazole (Terazol) should be considered. Single-dose oral fluconazole should be avoided.

Management options for complicated or recurrent yeast vaginitis

Extend any 7-day regimen to 10 to 14 days
Eliminate use of nylon or tight-fitting clothing
Consider discontinuing oral contraceptives
Consider eating 8 oz yogurt (with Lactobacillus acidophilus culture) per day
Improve glycemic control in diabetic patients
For long-term suppression of recurrent vaginitis, use ketoconazole, 100 mg (½ of 200-mg tablet) qd for 6 months

---

   D. Recurrent infection is defined as more than four episodes per year. Suppressive therapy for 6 months is recommended after completion of 10 to 14 days of a standard regimen. Oral ketoconazole, 100 mg daily for 6 months, has been shown to reduce the recurrence rate to 5%. If the sexual partner has balanitis, topical therapy should be prescribed.
IV. **Trichomoniasis**
   A. Trichomoniasis is responsible for less than 25% of vaginal infections. The infection is caused by Trichomonas vaginalis, which is a sexually transmitted disease. Most men are asymptomatic.
   B. **Diagnosis**
      1. A copious, watery discharge is common, and some patients may notice an odor. Often few symptoms are present. Usually, the vulva

and vaginal mucosa are free of signs of inflammation. The discharge is thin and characterized by an elevated pH, usually 6 to 7. Occasionally, small punctate cervical hemorrhages with ulcerations (strawberry cervix) are found.

2. Microscopic examination of vaginal fluid mixed with saline solution ("wet prep") shows an increased number of leukocytes and motile trichomonads. Microscopy has a sensitivity of only 50% to 70%. Trichomonads are sometimes reported on Pap smears, but false-positive results are common.

3. Culture for identification of T vaginalis has a sensitivity of 95% and should be performed when the clinical findings are consistent with trichomoniasis but motile organisms are absent. A rapid DNA probe test, which has a sensitivity of 90% and a specificity of 99.8%, can also be used.

C. **Treatment.** Oral metronidazole (Flagyl, Protostat) is recommended. Treatment of male sexual partners is recommended. Metronidazole gel (MetroGel-Vaginal) is less efficacious than oral antiinfective therapy. The single 2-g dose of oral metronidazole can be used safely in any trimester of pregnancy.

Treatment options for trichomoniasis

Initial measures
Metronidazole (Flagyl, Protostat), 2 g PO in a single dose, or metronidazole, 500 mg PO bid X 7 days, or metronidazole, 375 mg PO bid X 7 days
Treat male sexual partners

Measures for treatment failure
Treatment sexual contacts
Re-treat with metronidazole, 500 mg PO bid X 7 days
If infection persists, confirm with culture and re-treat with metronidazole, 2-4 g PO qd X 3-10 days

---

V. Bacterial Vaginosis

A. Bacterial vaginosis is a polymicrobial infection caused by an overgrowth of anaerobic organisms. It is the most common cause of vaginitis, accounting for 50% of cases. Gardnerella vaginalis has been identified as one of the key organisms in bacterial vaginosis.

B. **Diagnosis**

1. Most have vaginal discharge (90%) and foul odor (70%). Typically there is a homogeneous vaginal discharge, pH higher than 4.5, "clue cells" (epithelial cells studded with coccobacilli on microscopic examination, and a positive "whiff" test.

2. A specimen of vaginal discharge is obtained by speculum, and the pH is determined before the specimen is diluted. Next, the "whiff" test is performed by adding several drops of 10% KOH to the specimen. The test is positive when a fishy odor is detected. Finally, the specimen is viewed by wet-mount microscopy.

C. Treatment consists of oral metronidazole, 500 mg twice a day for 7 days. Common side effects of metronidazole include nausea, anorexia, abdominal cramps, and a metallic taste. Alcohol may cause a disulfiram-like reaction. Use of single-dose metronidazole may result in a higher recurrence rate and an increase in gastrointestinal side effects. Topical clindamycin is an option, but the cream may weaken latex condoms and diaphragms.

VI. Other diagnoses causing vaginal symptoms

A. One-third of patients with vaginal symptoms will not have laboratory evidence of bacterial vaginosis, Candida, or Trichomonas. Other causes of the vaginal symptoms include cervicitis, allergic reactions, and vulvodynia.

B. **Atrophic vaginitis** should be considered in postmenopausal patients if the mucosa appears pale and thin and wet-mount findings are negative.

1. **Oral estrogen (Premarin)** 0.3 mg qd should provide relief.
2. **Vaginal ring estradiol (Estring)**, a silastic ring impregnated with estradiol, is the preferred means of delivering estrogen to the vagina. The silastic ring delivers 6 to 9 μg of estradiol to the vagina daily. The rings are changed once every three months. Concomitant progestin therapy is not necessary.
3. **Conjugated estrogens (Premarin)**, 0.5 gm of cream, or one-eighth of an applicatorful daily into the vagina for three weeks, followed by twice weekly thereafter. Concomitant progestin therapy is not necessary.
4. **Estrace cream (estradiol)** can also by given by vaginal applicator at a dose of one-eighth of an applicator or 0.5 g (which contains 50 μg of estradiol) daily into the vagina for three weeks, followed by twice weekly thereafter. Concomitant progestin therapy is not necessary.

C. **Allergy and chemical irritation**
   1. Patients should be questioned about use of substances that cause allergic or chemical irritation, such as deodorant soaps, laundry detergent, vaginal contraceptives, bath oils, perfumed or dyed toilet paper, hot tub or swimming pool chemicals, and synthetic clothing.
   2. Topical steroids and systemic antihistamines can help alleviate the symptoms.

References: See page 166.

Gynecologic Oncology

Cervical Cancer

Invasive cervical carcinoma is the third most common cancer in the United States. The International Federation of Gynecology and Obstetrics (FIGO) recently revised its staging criteria. Survival rates for women with cervical cancer improve when radiotherapy is combined with cisplatin-based chemotherapy.

I. **Clinical evaluation**
  A. Human papillomavirus is the most important factor contributing to the development of cervical intraepithelial neoplasia and cervical cancer. Other epidemiologic risk factors associated with cervical intraepithelial neoplasia and cervical cancer include history of sexual intercourse at an early age, multiple sexual partners, sexually transmitted diseases (including chlamydia), and smoking. Additional risk factors include a male partner or partners who have had multiple sexual partners; previous history of squamous dysplasias of the cervix, vagina, or vulva; and immunosuppression.
  B. The signs and symptoms of early cervical carcinoma include watery vaginal discharge, intermittent spotting, and postcoital bleeding. Diagnosis often can be made with cytologic screening, colposcopically directed biopsy, or biopsy of a gross or palpable lesion. In cases of suspected microinvasion and early-stage cervical carcinoma, cone biopsy of the cervix is indicated to evaluate the possibility of invasion or to define the depth and extent of microinvasion. Cold knife cone biopsy provides the most accurate evaluation of the margins.
  C. **Histology.** The two major histologic types of invasive cervical carcinomas are squamous cell carcinomas and adenocarcinomas. Squamous cell carcinomas comprise 80% of cases, and adenocarcinoma or adenosquamous carcinoma comprise approximately 15%.

II. **Management**
  A. Early carcinomas of the cervix usually can be managed by surgical techniques or radiation therapy. The more advanced carcinomas require primary treatment with radiation therapy.
  B. **Staging of cervical carcinoma**
    1. Staging of invasive cervical cancer with the FIGO system is achieved by clinical evaluation.
    2. Careful clinical examination should be performed on all patients.
    3. Various optional examinations, such as ultrasonography, computed tomography (CT), magnetic resonance imaging (MRI), lymphangiography, laparoscopy, and fine-needle aspiration, are valuable for treatment planning. Surgical findings provide extremely accurate information about the extent of disease and will guide treatment plans but will not change the results of clinical staging.
    4. While not required as part of FIGO staging procedures, various radiologic tests are frequently undertaken to help define the extent of tumor growth and guide therapy decisions, especially in patients with locally advanced disease (ie, stage !!b or more advanced). Computed tomography of the abdomen and pelvis is the most widely used imaging study. MRI is as accurate as CT in assessing nodal involvement and provides better definition of the extent of local tumors within the pelvis.

Pretreatment Assessment of Women with Histologic Diagnosis of Cervical Cancer

History
Physical examination
Complete blood count, blood urea nitrogen, creatinine, hepatic function
Chest radiography
Intravenous pyelography or computed tomography of abdomen with intravenous contrast
Consider the following: barium enema, cystoscopy, rectosigmoidoscopy

Staging of Carcinoma of the Cervix Uteri: FIGO Nomenclature

Stage 0 Carcinoma in situ, cervical intraepithelial neoplasia Grade III

Stage I The carcinoma is strictly confined to the cervix (extension to the corpus would be disregarded).

Ia Invasive carcinoma that can be diagnosed only by microscopy. All macroscopically visible lesions-even with superficial invasion-are allotted to Stage Ib carcinomas. Invasion is limited to a measured stromal invasion with a maximal depth of 5.0 mm and a horizontal extension of not more than 7.0 mm. Depth of invasion should not be more than 5.0 mm taken from the base of the epithelium of the original tissue-superficial or glandular. The involvement of vascular spaces-venous or lymphatic-should not change the stage allotment.

   Ia1 Measured stromal invasion of not more than 3.0 mm in depth and extension of not more than 7.0 mm

   Ia2 Measured stromal invasion of more than 3.0 mm and not more than 5.0 mm with an extension of not more than 7.0 mm

Ib Clinically visible lesions limited to the cervix uteri or preclinical cancers greater than Stage Ia

   Ib1 Clinically visible lesions not more than 4.0 cm

   Ib2 Clinically visible lesions more than 4.0 cm

Stage II Cervical carcinoma invades beyond the uterus, but not to the pelvic wall or to the lower third of the vagina

IIa No obvious parametrial involvement

IIb Obvious parametrial involvement

Stage III The carcinoma has extended to the pelvic wall. On rectal examination, there is no cancer-free space between the tumor and the pelvic wall. The tumor involves the lower third of the vagina. All cases with hydronephrosis or nonfunctioning kidney are included, unless they are known to be due to other causes.

IIIa Tumor involves lower third of the vagina, with no extension to the pelvic wall

IIIb Extension to the pelvic wall or hydronephrosis or nonfunctioning kidney

Stage IV The carcinoma has extended beyond the true pelvis, or has involved (biopsy proved) the mucosa of the bladder or rectum. Bullous edema, as such, does not permit a case to be allotted to Stage IV.

IVa Spread of the growth to adjacent organs (bladder or rectum or both)

IVb Spread to distant organs

Guidelines for Clinical Staging of Invasive Cervical Carcinoma

Examinations should include inspection, palpation, colposcopy, endocervical curettage, hysteroscopy, cystoscopy, proctoscopy, intravenous pyelography, and X-ray examination of lungs and skeleton.

Conization of the cervix is considered a clinical examination.

Suspected bladder or rectal involvement should be confirmed histologically.

If there is a question about the most appropriate stage, the earlier stage should be assigned.

C. **Surgical evaluation of cervical carcinoma**. The results of surgical evaluation should not influence the stage determined by using the FIGO clinical staging system. However, the presence of lymph node metastasis is the most important adverse predictor of survival. Surgical evaluation of cervical cancer is the best method of assessing nodal involvement. Retroperitoneal surgical lymph node dissection of the pelvic and paraaortic lymph nodes provides important information about treatment planning and prognosis. Resection of positive lymph nodes is thought to provide therapeutic benefit.

D. **Treatment of microinvasive cervical cancer**. According to the FIGO criteria, patients with stage Ia 1 carcinoma could be treated with simple hysterectomy without nodal dissection or conization in selected cases. Those patients with invasion greater than 3 mm and no greater than 5 mm (stage Ia2) should undergo radical hysterectomy and pelvic lymphadenectomy. Although lymphatic-vascular invasion should not alter the FIGO stage, it is an important factor in treatment decisions. The risk of recurrence with lymphatic-vascular involvement is 3.1% if the extent of invasion is 3 mm or less and 15.7% if it is greater than 3 mm and no greater than 5 mm. Therefore, the presence of lymphatic-vascular invasion would suggest the need for more radical treatment.

E. **Treatment of early-stage (Ib-IIa) carcinoma**
   1. Both treatment strategies for stage Ib and early-stage IIa invasive carcinoma include 1) a primary surgical approach with radical hysterectomy and pelvic lymphadenectomy or 2) primary radiation therapy with external beam radiation and either high-dose-rate or low-dose-rate brachytherapy. The 5-year survival rate is 87-92% using either approach.
   2. Radical surgery leaves the vagina in more functional condition, while radiation therapy results in a reduction in length, caliber, and lubrication of the vagina. In premenopausal women, ovarian function can be preserved with surgery. The surgical approach also provides the opportunity for pelvic and abdominal exploration and provides better clinical and pathologic information with which to individualize treatment.

F. **Adjuvant therapy following primary surgery in early-stage carcinoma**
   1. Patients with histologically documented extracervical disease (pelvic nodal involvement, positive margins, or parametrial extension) are treated with concurrent pelvic radiation therapy and cisplatin-based chemotherapy. The use of combined adjuvant chemotherapy and radiation therapy in these high-risk patients following primary surgery significantly improves relapse-free survival and overall survival rates when compared with radiation therapy alone.
   2. Following radical hysterectomy, a subset of node-negative patients who have a constellation of primary risk factors (large tumors, depth of stromal infiltration, and lymphovascular space involvement) may be defined as having intermediate risk for relapse. For these patients, adjuvant pelvic radiation therapy provides clear therapeutic benefit,

with significantly improved relapse-free survival rates when compared with those who had no further therapy.

G. **Treatment of late-stage carcinoma (IIb or later)**. Cisplatin is usually administered weekly as a single agent because of its ease of delivery and favorable toxicity profile. Women with locally advanced cervical cancer in North America should receive cisplatin-based chemotherapy concurrent with radiation therapy.

H. **Long term monitoring**. Approximately 35% of patients will have persistent or recurrent disease. A common approach includes examinations and Pap tests every 3-4 months for the first 3 years, decreasing to twice yearly in the fourth and fifth years, with and chest X-rays annually for up to 5 years.

References: See page 166.

Endometrial Cancer

Uterine cancer is the most common malignant neoplasm of the female genital tract and the fourth most common cancer in women. About 6,000 women in the United States die of this disease each year. It is more frequent in affluent and white, especially obese, postmenopausal women of low parity. Hypertension and diabetes mellitus are also predisposing factors.

I. **Risk factors**

A. Any characteristic that increases exposure to unopposed estrogen increases the risk for endometrial cancer. Conversely, decreasing exposure to estrogen limits the risk. Unopposed estrogen therapy, obesity, anovulatory cycles and estrogen-secreting neoplasms all increase the amount of unopposed estrogen and thereby increase the risk for endometrial cancer. Smoking seems to decrease estrogen exposure, thereby decreasing the cancer risk, and oral contraceptive use increases progestin levels, thus providing protection.

B. **Hormone replacement therapy.** Unopposed estrogen treatment of menopause is associated with an eightfold increased incidence of endometrial cancer. The addition of progestin decreases this risk dramatically.

Risk Factors for Endometrial Cancer

Unopposed estrogen exposure
Median age at diagnosis: 59 years
Menstrual cycle irregularities, specifically menorrhagia and menometrorrhagia
Postmenopausal bleeding
Chronic anovulation
Nulliparity
Early menarche (before 12 years of age)
Late menopause (after 52 years of age)
Infertility
Tamoxifen (Nolvadex) use
Granulosa and thecal cell tumors
Ovarian dysfunction
Obesity
Diabetes mellitus
Arterial hypertension with or without atherosclerotic heart disease
History of breast or colon cancer

II. **Clinical evaluation**

A. Ninety percent of patients with endometrial cancer have abnormal vaginal bleeding, usually presenting as menometrorrhagia in a perimenopausal woman or menstrual-like bleeding in a woman past menopause. Perimenopausal women relate a history of intermenstrual bleeding, excessive bleeding lasting longer than seven days or an interval of less than 21 days between menses. Heavy, prolonged bleeding in patients known to be at risk for anovulatory cycles should prompt histologic evaluation of the endometrium. The size, contour, mobility and position of the uterus should be noted.

B. Patients who report abnormal vaginal bleeding and have risk factors for endometrial cancer should have histologic evaluation of the endometrium. Premenopausal patients with amenorrhea for more than six to 12 months should be offered endometrial sampling, especially if they have risk factors associated with excessive estrogen exposure. Postmenopausal women with vaginal bleeding who either are not on hormonal replacement therapy or have been on therapy longer than six months should be evaluated by endometrial sampling.

C. **Endometrial sampling**

1. In-office sampling of the endometrial lining may be accomplished with a Novak or Kevorkian curet, the Pipelle endometrial-suction curet, or the Vabra aspirator. Before having an in-office biopsy, the patient should take a preoperative dose of a nonsteroidal anti-inflammatory drug (NSAID). With the patient in the lithotomy position, a speculum is inserted in the vaginal canal. The cervix should be cleansed with a small amount of an antiseptic solution. After 1 mL of a local anesthetic is infused into the anterior lip of the cervix, a tenaculum is placed. The paracervical block is then performed using 1 or 2 percent lidocaine (Xylocaine) without epinephrine.

2. The cannula is then placed in the uterus and placement is confirmed with the help of the centimeter markings along the cannula. The inner sleeve is then pulled back while the cannula is held within the cavity. This generates a vacuum in the cannula that can be used to collect endometrial tissue for diagnosis. Moving the cannula in and out of the cavity no more than 2 to 3 cm with each stroke while turning the cannula clockwise or counterclockwise is helpful in obtaining specimens from the entire cavity.

III. **Treatment of endometrial cancer**

A. The treatment of endometrial cancer is usually surgical, such as total abdominal hysterectomy, bilateral salpingo-oophorectomy and evaluation for metastatic disease, which may include pelvic or para-aortic lymphadenectomy, peritoneal cytologic examination and peritoneal biopsies. The extent of the surgical procedure is based on the stage of disease, which can be determined only at the time of the operation.

Staging for Carcinoma of the Corpus Uteri	
Stage*	**Description**
IA (G1, G2, G3)	Tumor limited to endometrium
IB (G1, G2, G3)	Invasion of less than one half of the myometrium
IC (G1, G2, G3)	Invasion of more than one half of the myometrium
IIA (G1, G2, G3)	Endocervical gland involvement
IIB (G1, G2, G3)	Cervical stromal involvement
IIIA (G1, G2, G3)	Invasion of serosa and/or adnexa and/or positive peritoneal cytologic results
IIIB (G1, G2, G3)	Metastases to vagina

Stage*	Description
IIIC (G1, G2, G3)	Metastases to pelvic and/or para-aortic lymph nodes
IVA (G1, G2, G3)	Invasion of bladder and/or bowel mucosa
IVB	Distant metastases including intra-abdominal and/or inguinal lymph nodes

*--Carcinoma of the corpus is graded (G) according to the degree of histologic differentiation: G1 = 5 percent or less of a solid growth pattern; G2 = 6 to 50 percent of a solid growth pattern; G3 = more than 50 percent of a solid growth pattern.

    B. For most patients whose cancers have progressed beyond stage IB grade 2, postoperative radiation therapy is recommended. Because tumor response to cytotoxic chemotherapy has been poor, chemotherapy is used only for palliation.

    C. Endometrial hyperplasia with atypia should be treated with hysterectomy except in extraordinary cases. Progestin treatment is a possibility in women younger than 40 years of age who refuse hysterectomy or who wish to retain their childbearing potential, but an endometrial biopsy should be performed every three months. Treatment of atypical hyperplasia and well-differentiated endometrial cancer with progestins in women younger than 40 years of age results in complete regression of disease in 94 percent and 75 percent, respectively.

    D. Patients found to have hyperplasia without atypia should be treated with progestins and have an endometrial biopsy every three to six months.

IV. Serous and clear cell adenocarcinomas

    A. These cancers are considered in a separate category from endometrioid adenocarcinomas. They have a worse prognosis overall. Patients with serous carcinomas have a poorer survival. The 3 year survival is 40% for stage I disease.

    B. Serous and clear cell carcinomas are staged like ovarian cancer. A total abdominal hysterectomy and bilateral salpingo-oophorectomy, lymph node biopsy, and omental biopsy/omentectomy are completed. Washings from the pelvis, gutters and diaphragm are obtained, and the diaphragm is sampled and peritoneal biopsies completed.

References: See page 166.

Ovarian Cancer

A woman has a 1-in-70 risk of developing ovarian cancer in her lifetime. The incidence is 1.4 per 100,000 women under age 40, increasing to approximately 45 per 100,000 for women over age 60. The median age at diagnosis is 61. A higher incidence of ovarian cancer is seen in women who have never been pregnant or who are of low parity. Women who have had either breast or colon cancer or have a family history of these cancers also are at higher risk of developing ovarian cancer. Protective factors include multiparity, oral contraceptive use, a history of breastfeeding, and anovulatory disorders.

I. Screening. There is no proven method of screening for ovarian cancer. Routine screening by abdominal or vaginal ultrasound or measurement of CA 125 levels in serum cannot be recommended for women with no known risk factors. For women with familial ovarian cancer syndrome who wish to maintain their reproductive capacity, transvaginal ultrasonography, analysis of levels of CA 125 in serum, or both, in combination with frequent pelvic examinations may be considered.

II. Diagnosis

   A. History. There are no early symptoms of cancer of the ovary. Abdominal discomfort, upper abdominal fullness, and early satiety are associated with cancer of the ovary. Other frequently encountered signs and symptoms are fatigue, increasing abdominal girth, urinary frequency, and shortness of breath caused by pleural effusion or massive ascites.

   B. Physical findings. The most frequently noted physical finding of ovarian cancer is a pelvic mass. An adnexal mass that is bilateral, irregular, solid, or fixed suggests malignancy. Other findings suggestive of malignancy are ascites or a nodular cul-de-sac. The risk of ovarian cancer is significantly higher in premenarcheal and postmenopausal women with an adnexal mass than in women of reproductive age.

   C. Diagnostic workup

   1. Initial evaluation with a thorough history, physical examination, and vaginal probe ultrasonography will distinguish most benign masses from malignant masses. Chest X-ray is performed to rule out parenchymal or pleural involvement with effusion. Screening mammography, if it has not been done within 6-12 months, should be performed preoperatively to rule out another primary source.

   2. Other studies that may be helpful in the diagnostic workup include barium enema, upper gastrointestinal series, colonoscopy, upper gastrointestinal endoscopy, intravenous pyelography, and computed tomography (CT) scan or magnetic resonance imaging.

   3. The tumor marker CA 125 may assist in evaluation. Sustained elevation of CA 125 levels occurs in more than 80% of patients with nonmucinous epithelial ovarian carcinomas but in only 1% of the general population. Levels of CA 125 in serum also may be elevated in patients with conditions such as endometriosis, leiomyomata, pelvic inflammatory disease, hepatitis, congestive heart failure, cirrhosis, and malignancies other than ovarian carcinomas. In postmenopausal patients with pelvic masses, CA 125 levels in serum greater than 65 U/mL are predictive of a malignancy in 75% of cases.

III. Primary treatment of epithelial ovarian cancer

   A. Primary therapy for ovarian cancer is complete staging and optimal reduction of tumor volume. Subsequent therapy depends on the operative findings.

   B. Staging

   1. Ovarian cancer staging is based on surgical evaluation. Accurate staging is of utmost importance for planning further therapy and in discussing prognosis. Staging is determined by clinical, surgical, histologic, and pathologic findings, including results of cytologic testing of effusions or peritoneal washings. Pleural effusions should be sampled.

   2. **Operative techniques**

      a. The incision used should provide maximum exposure of the pelvis and allow thorough evaluation of the upper abdomen. If present, ascites should be aspirated and sent for cytopathologic evaluation. A small amount of heparin should be added to prevent clotting of bloody or mucoid specimens. If ascites is not present, abdominal washings with saline should be obtained from the pericolic gutters, the suprahepatic space, and the pelvis. A Pap test of the diaphragm should be taken.

      b. The abdominal cavity should be explored systematically. The lower surface of the diaphragm, the upper abdominal recesses, the liver, and retroperitoneal nodes should be carefully noted for tumor involvement. In addition, the intestines, mesentery, and omentum should be examined. The presence or absence of metastases in the pelvis and abdomen should be noted, and the exact location and size of tumor nodules should be described.

      c. In cases in which disease is grossly confined to the pelvis, efforts should be made to detect occult metastasis with peritoneal cytologies, biopsies of peritoneum from the pelvis and pericolic gutters, and resection of the greater omentum. In addition, selective pelvic and paraaortic lymphadenectomy also should be carried out.

Definitions of the Stages in Primary Carcinoma of the Ovary	
Stage	**Definition**
I	Growth is limited to the ovaries
IA	Growth is limited to one ovary; no ascites present containing malignant cells; no tumor on the external surface; capsule is intact
IB	Growth is limited to both ovaries; no ascites present containing malignant cells; no tumor on the external surfaces; capsules are intact
IC	Tumor is classified as either stage IA or IB but with tumor on the surface of one or both ovaries; or with ruptured capsule(s); or with ascites containing malignant cells present or with positive peritoneal washings
II	Growth involves one or both ovaries with pelvic extension
IIA	Extension and/or metastases to the uterus and/or tubes
IIB	Extension to other pelvic tissues
IIC	Tumor is either stage IIA or IIb but with tumor on the surface of one or both ovaries; or with capsule(s) ruptured; or with ascites containing malignant cells present or with positive peritoneal washings
III	Tumor involves one or both ovaries with peritoneal implants outside the pelvis and/or positive retroperitoneal or inguinal nodes; superficial liver metastasis equals stage III; tumor is limited to the true pelvis but with histologically proven malignant extension to small bowel or omentum
IIIA	Tumor is grossly limited to the true pelvis with negative nodes but with histologically confirmed microscopic seeding of abdominal peritoneal surfaces
IIIB	Tumor involves one or both ovaries with histologically confirmed implants of abdominal peritoneal surfaces, none exceeding 2 cm in diameter; nodes are negative
IIIC	Abdominal implants greater than 2 cm in diameter and/or positive retroperitoneal or inguinal nodes
IV	Growth involves one or both ovaries with distant metastases; if pleural effusion is present, there must be positive cytology findings to assign a case to stage IV; parenchymal liver metastasis equals stage IV

C. **Cytoreductive surgery** improves response to chemotherapy and survival of women with advanced ovarian cancer. Operative management is designed to remove as much tumor as possible. When a malignant tumor is present, a thorough abdominal exploration, total abdominal hysterectomy, bilateral salpingo-oophorectomy, lymphadenectomy, omentectomy, and removal of all gross cancer are standard therapy.

D. **Adjuvant therapy**
   1. Patients with stage IA or IB disease (who have been completely surgically staged) and who have borderline, well- or moderately differentiated tumors do not benefit from additional chemotherapy because their prognosis is excellent with surgery alone.
   2. Chemotherapy improves survival and is an effective means of palliation of ovarian cancer. In patients who are at increased risk of recurrence (stage I G3 and all IC-IV), chemotherapy is recommended.

Sequential clinical trials of chemotherapy agents demonstrate that cisplatin (or carboplatin) given in combination with paclitaxel is the most active combination identified.

References: See page 166.

Breast Cancer

One of 8 women will develop breast cancer. The risk of breast cancer increases with age; approximately half of new cases occur in women aged 65 years or older. Two percent of 40- to 49-year-old women in the United States develop breast cancer during the fifth decade of their lives, and 0.3% die from breast cancer. Breast cancer is the most common malignancy in American women, and the second most lethal malignancy in women, following lung cancer.

I. Risk Factors

A. Major risk factors for breast cancer include: 1) early menarche, 2) nulliparity, 3) delayed childbirth, 4) increasing age, 5) race, and 6) family history.

Risk Factors for Breast Cancer

Major Risk Factors
Early menarche
Nulliparity
Delayed childbirth
Increasing age
Race
Family history

Other Risk Factors

Late menopause	A history of breast cancer
Obesity	Exposure to ionizing radiation
Weight gain	Higher bone mineral density
Increased intra-abdominal fat (android body habitus)	Smoking
	Alcohol consumption
Lack of regular exercise	Elevated insulin-like growth factor- I
Elevated serum estradiol	(IGF- I) levels
Elevated free testosterone levels	Increased mammographic density
A previous premalignant breast biopsy	Oral contraceptives
Radial scars in benign breast biopsies	

Familial Risk Factors for Breast Cancer
More than 50% of women in family have breast cancer
Breast cancer present in more than I generation
Multiple occurrences of breast cancer (>3) in close relatives
Onset at less than age 45 years
History of bilateral breast cancer
High rate of co-existing ovarian cancer
BRCA1 gene mutation

B. Nulliparity and increased age at first pregnancy are associated with an increased risk for breast cancer. Nulliparity alone accounts for 16% of new cases of breast cancer each year. The relative risk for breast cancer increases with advancing age.

C. Race is an independent risk factor. While white women are at an increased risk for breast cancer, African American women with breast cancer have higher fatality rates and a later stage at diagnosis.

D. A family history of breast cancer, especially in first-degree relatives, increases the risk.

E. A history of breast cancer increases a woman's risk for subsequent breast cancers. If the woman has no family history of breast cancer, then the initial occurrence was sporadic, and the incidence for developing a second breast cancer is 1% per year. If the initial occurrence was hereditary, the incidence for developing a second breast cancer is 3% per year. Approximately 10% of women with breast cancer will develop a second primary breast cancer.

F. Familial or Genetic Risk Factors. A mutation in a tumor-suppresser gene occurs in 1 of 400 women and is located on chromosome 17q. Carriers of a BRCA1 mutation have an 85% lifetime risk of developing breast cancer. In addition, the risk of colon and ovarian cancers is also increased (40% to 50%) in these groups. The 70% of breast cancer patients who do not have inherited mutations on BRCA1 have mutations on BRCA2. The cumulative lifetime risk of breast cancer in a woman with the BRCA2 mutation is 87%.

G. Conclusions. Seventy-five percent of women with newly diagnosed breast cancer demonstrate no specific, identifiable risk factor. Most premenopausal breast cancer cases are genetically determined. In contrast, many post-menopausal cases are environmentally related.

II. Screening Guidelines

A. Breast Self-Examination. All women older than age 20 years should perform regular monthly breast self-examinations. Menstruating women should examine their breasts in the first 7 to 10 days of the menstrual cycle.

Breast Screening Criteria		
Age	Clinical Breast Examination	Mammography
30-39	Every 1-3 years	None
40-49	Annual	Optional 1-2 years
≥ 50	Annual	Annual
Women aged 50 to 69 years should be offered mammography and receive a clinical breast examination every 1 to 2 years.		

B. Clinical Breast Examination (CBE) is recommended every 1 to 3 years for women aged 30 to 39 years and annually for those aged 40 years and older.

C. Mammography. Mammography alone is 75% sensitive, and, when combined with CBE, the screening sensitivity for detecting breast cancer increases to 88%. Screening guidelines from the US Preventive Services Task Force suggest mammography alone or with CBE every 1 to 2 years for women aged 50 to 69 years. Recent evidence suggests a benefit from annual mammography with or without CBE for women aged 40 to 49 years.

III. History and Physical Examination

A. In the woman with a suspicious breast mass, risk factors and a family history of breast cancers should be assessed. A personal history of radiation to the chest or breast, breast masses, biopsies, history of collagen vascular disease, and menstrual and gynecologic history are also important. Symptoms of nipple discharge, pain, skin changes, or rashes may occur.

B. On physical examination, the breast mass should be palpated for size, position, adherence of the tumor to the skin or chest wall, density, fluctuance, and tenderness. In addition, both breasts and axillae should be examined for other tumors and any lymph nodes. A search for supraclavicular lymph nodes should also be conducted.

C. Any evidence of skin changes, ulceration, peau d'orange (thickening of skin to resemble an orange skin), or lymphedema is suspicious for locally advanced cancer.

    D. Immediate mammography should be obtained. A white blood count, hematocrit, and erythrocyte sedimentation rate may be needed if cancer is found.

IV. Diagnosis

    A. The definitive diagnosis is made by pathological evaluation of tissue.

    B. A combination of clinical breast examination, mammography, and fine-needle aspiration and biopsy may be sufficient to make a diagnosis. If all studies are "benign," there is a greater than 99% chance that a benign breast lesion is present.

    C. Open biopsy in the operating room or wire-localization of a suspicious lesion noted on mammography may be necessary if fine-needle aspiration and biopsy is nondiagnostic. Biopsy by stereo-tactic technique in radiology also may be used to obtain tissue for diagnosis of the suspicious area.

V. Definition and classification of breast cancer for staging

    A. The definition for staging and the classification of stages for breast cancer follow the system of the International Union Against Cancer. This system is based on the tumor, nodes, and metastases (TNM) nomenclature.

Definitions for Breast Cancer Staging	
Tumor	
TIS	Carcinoma in situ (intraductal carcinoma, lobular)
T0	No evidence of primary tumor
T1	Tumor ≤2 cm in greatest dimension
T2	Tumor >2 cm but <5 cm in greatest dimension
T3	Tumor >5 cm in greatest dimension
T4	Tumor of any size with direct extension into chest wall or skin
Nodes	
N0	No regional lymph node metastases
N1	Metastases to movable ipsilateral axillary node(s)
N2	Metastases to ipsilateral axillary lymph node(s), fixed to one another or other structures
Metastases	
M0	No distant metastases
M I	Metastases to movable ipsilateral axillary node(s); metastases to ipsilateral axillary lymph node(s); fixed to one another or other structures; or metastases to ipsilateral internal mammary lymph node(s); distant metastases

Classification of Breast Cancer Staging	
Stage	Description*
0	TIS, N0, M0
I	TI, N0, M0
IIA	T0, NI, M0
IIB	T2, NI, M0, or T3, N0, M0
IIIA	T0, N2, M0, or TI, N2, M0, or T2, N2, M0, or T3, NI, or N2, M0
IIIB	T4, any N, M0 or any T, N3
IV	Any T, any N, MI

*Tumor/nodes/metastases

- **B.** The HER-2 gene (c-erbB-2, HER-2/neu) has been identified, and the HER-2 receptor is correlated with aggressive biological behavior of the cancer and a poor clinical outcome.
- **C.** The staging of breast cancer dictates not only the prognosis but also directs treatment modality recommendations. The prognosis for women is based on their age, tumor type, initial tumor size, presence of nodes and staging, and hormone-re-ceptor status. The overall 10-year survival rates for the more common breast cancer stages are greater than 90% for stage 0, greater than 75% for stage I, greater than 50% for stage IIA, and approximately 50% for stage IIB.

VI. Treatment of breast cancer

- **A.** Treatment choices for ductal carcinoma in situ, a stage 0 cancer, include 1) mastectomy, 2) lumpectomy followed by radiation therapy, or 3) lumpectomy followed by radiation therapy and then tamoxifen if the tumor is estrogen-receptor test positive.
- **B. Surgical Treatment**
  1. Several long-term studies show that conservative therapy and radiation result in at least as good a prognosis as radical mastectomy. Skin-sparing mastectomy involves removing all the breast tissue, the nipple, and the areolar complex. The remainder of the surface skin tissue remains intact. Reconstruction is then completed with a natural-appearing breast. This procedure is considered for those women with ductal carcinoma in situ or T1 or T2 invasive carcinomas. Because a mastectomy leaves 3.5% of the breast tissue behind, the recurrence rate for this procedure is comparable with a modified radical mastectomy.
  2. Local excision of the tumor mass (lumpectomy) followed by lymph node staging and subsequent adjuvant hormone therapy, chemotherapy, or radiation therapy is an accepted treatment. Long-term studies have found that recurrence rates are similar when lumpectomy was compared with radiation therapy and mastectomy. One study showed no recurrence if 1-cm margins were obtained followed by the use of radiation therapy.
- **C. Radiation Therapy.** External beam radiation therapy has proven effective in preventing recurrence of breast cancer and for palliation of pain. The risk of relapse after radiation therapy ranges from 4% to 10%. Lumpectomy can now be performed followed by implantation of high-dose brachytherapy catheters.
- **D. Anti-Hormonal Therapy.** Hormonal therapy is indicated for those

tumors that test positive for hormone receptors. Tamoxifen has both estrogenic and anti-estrogenic effects. In women who are older than 50 years with breast cancers that test positive for hormone receptors, tamoxifen use produces a 20% increase in 5-year survival rates. The response rate in advanced cases increases to 35%.

E. Chemotherapy

1. Chemotherapy is used in women at risk for metastatic disease. Cytotoxic agents used include methotrexate, fluorouracil, cyclophosphamide (Cytoxan, Neosar), doxorubicin, mitoxantrone (Novantrone), and paclitaxel (Taxol). In the management of stage 0 disease, chemotherapy is not used initially.

2. Stage I and stage II disease are treated with chemotherapy based on the relative risk of systemic recurrence. This risk is often based on the woman's age, axillary lymph node involvement, tumor size, hormone receptor status, histologic tumor grade, and cellular aggressiveness. Systemic chemotherapy is recommended for women with stage I disease who have node-negative cancers and a tumor size greater than 1 cm in diameter.

3. Women with stage IIA breast cancer are treated with adjuvant chemotherapy with or without tamoxifen. Some women with positive lymph nodes are placed on chemotherapy, including doxorubicin, fluorouracil, and methotrexate.

4. In women with stage III breast cancer, similar agents are selected. Doxorubicin is particularly useful in treating inflammatory breast cancer. In women with stage IIIB cancer, chemotherapy is usually administered before primary surgery or radiation therapy. High-dose chemotherapy plus stem-cell transplantation does not improve survival rates. In women with stage IV disease, chemotherapy is useful in treating metastatic breast cancer.

References: See page 166.

Obstetrics

Prenatal Care

I. **Prenatal history and physical examination**
   A. **Diagnosis of pregnancy**
   1. **Amenorrhea** is usually the first sign of conception. Other symptoms include breast fullness and tenderness, skin changes, nausea, vomiting, urinary frequency, and fatigue.
   2. **Pregnancy tests.** Urine pregnancy tests may be positive within days of the first missed menstrual period. Serum beta human chorionic gonadotropin (HCG) is accurate up to a few days after implantation.
   3. **Fetal heart tones** can be detected as early as 11-12 weeks from the last menstrual period (LMP) by Doppler. The normal fetal heart rate is 120-160 beats per minute.
   4. **Fetal movements** ("quickening") are first felt by the patient at 17-19 weeks.
   5. **Ultrasound** will visualize a gestational sac at 5-6 weeks and a fetal pole with movement and cardiac activity by 7-8 weeks. Ultrasound can estimate fetal age accurately if completed before 24 weeks.
   6. **Estimated date of confinement.** The mean duration of pregnancy is 40 weeks from the LMP. Estimated date of confinement (EDC) can be calculated by Nägele's rule: Add 7 days to the first day of the LMP, then subtract 3 months.
   B. **Contraceptive history.** Recent oral contraceptive usage often causes postpill amenorrhea, and may cause erroneous pregnancy dating.
   C. **Gynecologic and obstetric history**
   1. Gravidity is the total number of pregnancies. Parity is expressed as the number of term pregnancies, preterm pregnancies, abortions, and live births.
   2. The character and length of previous labors, type of delivery, complications, infant status, and birth weight are recorded.
   3. Assess prior cesarean sections and determine type of C-section (low transverse or classical), and determine reason it was performed.
   D. **Medical and surgical history** and prior hospitalizations are documented.
   E. **Medications** and allergies are recorded.
   F. **Family history** of medical illnesses, hereditary illness, or multiple gestation is sought.
   G. **Social history.** Cigarettes, alcohol, or illicit drug use.
   H. **Review of systems.** Abdominal pain, constipation, headaches, vaginal bleeding, dysuria or urinary frequency, or hemorrhoids.
   I. **Physical examination**
   1. Weight, funduscopic examination, thyroid, breast, lungs, and heart are examined.
   2. An extremity and neurologic exam are completed, and the presence of a cesarean section scar is sought.
   3. **Pelvic examination**
      a. Pap smear and culture for gonorrhea are completed routinely. Chlamydia culture is completed in high-risk patients.
      b. Estimation of gestational age by uterine size
         (1) The nongravid uterus is 3 x 4 x 7 cm. The uterus begins to change in size at 5-6 weeks.
         (2) Gestational age is estimated by uterine size: 8 weeks = 2 x normal size; 10 weeks = 3 x normal; 12 weeks = 4 x normal.
         (3) At 12 weeks the fundus becomes palpable at the symphysis pubis.
         (4) At 16 weeks, the uterus is midway between the symphysis pubis and the umbilicus.
         (5) At 20 weeks, the uterus is at the umbilicus. After 20 weeks,

there is a correlation between the number of weeks of gestation and the number of centimeters from the pubic symphysis to the top of the fundus.

(6) Uterine size that exceeds the gestational dating by 3 or more weeks suggests multiple gestation, molar pregnancy, or (most commonly) an inaccurate date for LMP. Ultrasonography will confirm inaccurate dating or intrauterine growth failure.

   c. Adnexa are palpated for masses.

II. Initial visit laboratory testing

A. CBC, AB blood typing and Rh factor, antibody screen, rubella, VDRL/RPR, hepatitis B surface Ag.

B. Pap smear, urine pregnancy test, urinalysis and urine culture. Cervical culture for gonorrhea and chlamydia.

C. Tuberculosis skin testing, HIV counseling/testing.

D. Hemoglobin electrophoresis is indicated in risks groups, such as sickle hemoglobin in African patients, B-thalassemia in Mediterranean patients, and alpha-thalassemia in Asian patients. Tay-Sachs carrier testing is indicated in Jewish patients.

III. Clinical assessment at first trimester prenatal visits

A. Assessment at each prenatal visit includes maternal weight, blood pressure, uterine size, and evaluation for edema, proteinuria, and glucosuria.

B. First Doppler heart tones should become detectable at 10-12 weeks, and they should be sought thereafter.

C. Routine prenatal vitamins are probably not necessary. Folic acid supplementation preconceptually and throughout the early part of pregnancy has been shown to decrease the incidence of fetal neural tube defects.

Frequency of Prenatal Care Visits in Low-Risk Pregnancies	
<28 weeks	Every month
28-36 weeks	Every 2 weeks
36-delivery	Every 1 week until delivery

D. **First Trimester Education.** Discuss smoking, alcohol, exercise, diet, and sexuality.

E. **Headache and backache.** Acetaminophen (Tylenol) 325-650 mg every 3-4 hours is effective. Aspirin is contraindicated.

F. **Nausea and vomiting.** First-trimester morning sickness may be relieved by eating frequent, small meals, getting out of bed slowly after eating a few crackers, and by avoiding spicy or greasy foods. Promethazine (Phenergan) 12.5-50 mg PO q4-6h prn or diphenhydramine (Benadryl) 25-50 mg tid-qid is useful.

G. **Constipation.** A high-fiber diet with psyllium (Metamucil), increased fluid intake, and regular exercise should be advised. Docusate (Colace) 100 mg bid may provide relief.

IV. Clinical assessment at second trimester visits

A. Questions for each follow-up visit

1. **First detection of fetal movement (quickening)** should occur at around 17 weeks in a multigravida and at 19 weeks in a primigravida. **Fetal movement** should be documented at each visit after 17 weeks.

2. **Vaginal bleeding or symptoms of preterm labor** should be sought.

B. **Fetal heart rate** is documented at each visit

C. **Maternal serum testing at 15-16 weeks**

1. **Triple screen** (α-fetoprotein, human chorionic gonadotropin [hCG], and estriol). In women under age 35 years, screening for fetal Down syndrome is accomplished with a triple screen. Maternal serum alpha-fetoprotein is elevated in 20-25% of all cases of Down syndrome, and it is elevated in fetal neural tube deficits. Levels of hCG are higher in

Down syndrome and levels of unconjugated estriol are lower in Down syndrome.
   2. If levels are abnormal, an ultrasound examination is performed and genetic amniocentesis is offered. The triple screen identifies 60% of Down syndrome cases. Low levels of all three serum analytes identifies 60-75% of all cases of fetal trisomy 18.
   D. **At 15-18 weeks, genetic amniocentesis** should be offered to patients ≥35 years old, and it should be offered if a birth defect has occurred in the mother, father, or in previous offspring.
   E. **Screening ultrasound** should usually be obtained at 16-18 weeks.
   F. **At 24-28 weeks,** a one-hour Glucola (blood glucose measurement 1 hour after 50-gm oral glucose) is obtained to screen for gestational diabetes. Those with a particular risk (eg, previous gestational diabetes or fetal macrosomia), require earlier testing. If the 1 hour test result is greater than 140 mg/dL, a 3-hour glucose tolerance test is necessary.
   G. **Second trimester education.** Discomforts include backache, round ligament pain, constipation, and indigestion.
V. **Clinical assessment at third trimester visits**
   A. **Fetal movement** is documented. Vaginal bleeding or symptoms of preterm labor should be sought. Preeclampsia symptoms (blurred vision, headache, rapid weight gain, edema) are sought.
   B. **Fetal heart rate** is documented at each visit.
   C. **At 26-30 weeks,** repeat hemoglobin and hematocrit are obtained to determine the need for iron supplementation.
   D. **At 28-30 weeks,** an antibody screen is obtained in Rh-negative women, and D immune globulin (RhoGAM) is administered if negative.
   E. **At 36 weeks,** repeat serologic testing for syphilis is recommended for high risk groups.
   F. **Gonorrhea and chlamydia screening is repeated** in the third-trimester in high-risk patients.
   G. **Screening for group B streptococcus colonization at 35-37 weeks**
      1. Lower vaginal and rectal cultures are recommended; cultures should not be collected by speculum examination. The optimal method for GBS screening is collection of a single standard culture swab of the distal vagina and rectum.
   H. **Third trimester education**
      1. **Signs of labor.** The patient should call physician when rupture of membranes or contractions have occurred every 5 minutes for one hour.
      2. **Danger signs.** Preterm labor, rupture of membranes, bleeding, edema, signs of preeclampsia.
      3. **Common discomforts.** Cramps, edema, frequent urination.
   I. **At 36 weeks,** a cervical exam may be completed. Fetal position should be assessed by palpation (Leopold's Maneuvers).
References: See page 166.

Normal Labor

Labor consists of the process by which uterine contractions expel the fetus. A term pregnancy is 37 to 42 weeks from the last menstrual period (LMP).

I. **Obstetrical History and Physical Examination**
   A. **History of the present labor**
      1. **Contractions.** The frequency, duration, onset, and intensity of uterine contractions should be determined. Contractions may be accompanied by a "bloody show" (passage of blood-tinged mucus from the dilating cervical os). Braxton Hicks contractions are often felt by patients during the last weeks of pregnancy. They are usually irregular, mild, and do not cause cervical change.
      2. **Rupture of membranes.** Leakage of fluid may occur alone or in

conjunction with uterine contractions. The patient may report a large gush of fluid or increased moisture. The color of the liquid should be determine, including the presence of blood or meconium.
3. **Vaginal bleeding** should be assessed. Spotting or blood-tinged mucus is common in normal labor. Heavy vaginal bleeding may be a sign of placental abruption.
4. **Fetal movement.** A progressive decrease in fetal movement from baseline, should prompt an assessment of fetal well-being with a nonstress test or biophysical profile.

B. **History of present pregnancy**
1. **Estimated date of confinement** (EDC) is calculated as 40 weeks from the first day of the LMP.
2. **Fetal heart tones** are first heard with a Doppler instrument 10-12 weeks from the LMP.
3. **Quickening** (maternal perception of fetal movement) occurs at about 17 weeks.
4. **Uterine size** before 16 weeks is an accurate measure of dates.
5. **Ultrasound** measurement of fetal size before 24 weeks of gestation is an accurate measure of dates.
6. **Prenatal history**. Medical problems during this pregnancy should be reviewed, including urinary tract infections, diabetes, or hypertension.
7. **Antepartum testing.** Nonstress tests, contraction stress tests, biophysical profiles.
8. **Review of systems.** Severe headaches, scotomas, hand and facial edema, or epigastric pain (preeclampsia) should be sought. Dysuria, urinary frequency or flank pain may indicate cystitis or pyelonephritis.

C. **Obstetrical history.** Past pregnancies, durations and outcomes, preterm deliveries, operative deliveries, prolonged labors, pregnancy-induced hypertension should be assessed.

D. **Past medical history** of asthma, hypertension, or renal disease should be sought.

II. **Physical examination**
A. Vital signs are assessed.
B. **Head.** Funduscopy should seek hemorrhages or exudates, which may suggest diabetes or hypertension. Facial, hand and ankle edema suggest preeclampsia.
C. **Chest.** Auscultation of the lungs for wheezes and crackles may indicate asthma or heart failure.
D. **Uterine Size.** Until the middle of the third trimester, the distance in centimeters from the pubic symphysis to the uterine fundus should correlate with the gestational age in weeks. Toward term, the measurement becomes progressively less reliable because of engagement of the presenting part.
E. **Estimation of fetal weight** is completed by palpation of the gravid uterus.
F. **Leopold's maneuvers** are used to determine the position of the fetus.
1. **The first maneuver** determines which fetal pole occupies the uterine fundus. The breech moves with the fetal body. The vertex is rounder and harder, feels more globular than the breech, and can be moved separately from the fetal body.
2. **Second maneuver.** The lateral aspects of the uterus are palpated to determine on which side the fetal back or fetal extremities (the small parts) are located.
3. **Third maneuver.** The presenting part is moved from side to side. If movement is difficult, engagement of the presenting part has occurred.
4. **Fourth maneuver.** With the fetus presenting by vertex, the cephalic prominence may be palpable on the side of the fetal small parts.
G. **Pelvic examination.** The adequacy of the bony pelvis, the integrity of the fetal membranes, the degree of cervical dilatation and effacement, and the station of the presenting part should be determined.
H. **Extremities.** Severe lower extremity or hand edema suggests preeclampsia. Deep-tendon hyperreflexia and clonus may signal

impending seizures.
  I. **Laboratory tests**
     1. Prenatal labs should be documented, including CBC, blood type, Rh, antibody screen, serologic test for syphilis, rubella antibody titer, urinalysis, culture, Pap smear, cervical cultures for gonorrhea and Chlamydia, and hepatitis B surface antigen (HbsAg).
     2. During labor, the CBC, urinalysis and RPR are repeated. The HBSAG is repeated for high-risk patients. A clot of blood is placed on hold.
  J. **Fetal heart rate.** The baseline heart rate, variability, accelerations, and decelerations are recorded.

Labor History and Physical

Chief compliant: Contractions, rupture of membranes.
HPI: ___ year old Gravida (number of pregnancies) Para (number of deliveries).
Gestational age, last menstrual period, estimated date of confinement.
Contractions (onset, frequency, intensity), rupture of membranes (time, color). Vaginal bleeding (consistency, quantity, bloody show); fetal movement.
Fetal Heart Rate Strip: Baseline rate, accelerations, reactivity, decelerations, contraction frequency.
Dates: First day of last menstrual period, estimated date of confinement. Ultrasound dating.
Prenatal Care: Date of first exam, number of visits; has size been equal to dates? infections, hypertension, diabetes.
Obstetrical History: Dates of prior pregnancies, gestational age, route (C-section with indications and type of uterine incision), weight, complications, length of labor, hypertension.
Gynecologic History: Menstrual history (menarche, interval, duration), herpes, gonorrhea, chlamydia, abortions; oral contraceptives.
Past Medical History: Illnesses, asthma, hypertension, diabetes, renal disease, surgeries.
Medications: Iron, prenatal vitamins.
Allergies: Penicillin, codeine?
Social History: Smoking, alcohol, drug use.
Family History: Hypertension, diabetes, bleeding disorders.
Review of Systems: Severe headaches, scotomas, blurred vision, hand and face edema, epigastric pain, pruritus, dysuria, fever.

Physical Exam
General Appearance:
Vitals: BP, pulse, respirations, temperature.
HEENT: Funduscopy, facial edema, jugular venous distention.
Chest: Wheezes, rhonchi.
Cardiovascular: Rhythm, S1, S2, murmurs.
Abdomen: Fundal height, Leopold's maneuvers (lie, presentation). Estimated fetal weight (EFW), tenderness, scars.
Cervix: Dilatation, effacement, station, position, status of membranes, presentation. Vulvar herpes lesions.
Extremities: Cyanosis, clubbing, edema.
Neurologic: Deep tender reflexes, clonus.
Prenatal Labs: Obtain results of one hour post glucola, RPR/VDRL, rubella, blood type, Rh, CBC, Pap, PPD, hepatitis BsAg, UA, C and S.
Current Labs: Hemoglobin, hematocrit, glucose, UA; urine dipstick for protein.
Assessment: Intrauterine pregnancy (IUP) at 40 weeks, admitted with the following problems:
Plan: Anticipated type of labor and delivery. List plan for each problem.

III. **Normal labor**
   A. Labor is characterized by uterine contractions of sufficient frequency, intensity, and duration to result in effacement and dilatation of the cervix.
   B. **The first stage of labor** starts with the onset of regular contractions and ends with complete dilatation (10 cm). This stage is further subdivided into the latent and an active phases.
      1. The latent phase starts with the onset of regular uterine contractions and is characterized by slow cervical dilatation to 4 cm. The latent phase is variable in length.
      2. The active phase follows and is characterized by more rapid dilatation to 10 cm. During the active phase of labor, the average rate of cervical dilatation is 1.5 cm/hour in the multipara and 1.2 cm/hour in the nullipara.
   C. **The second stage of labor** begins with complete dilatation of the cervix and ends with delivery of the infant. It is characterized by voluntary and involuntary pushing. The average second stage of labor is one-half hour in a multipara and 1 hour in the primipara.
   D. **The third stage of labor** begins with the delivery of the infant and ends with the delivery of the placenta.
   E. **Intravenous fluids**. IV fluid during labor is usually Ringer's lactate or 0.45% normal saline with 5% dextrose. Intravenous fluid infused rapidly or given as a bolus should be dextrose-free because maternal hyperglycemia can occur.
   F. **Activity.** Patients in the latent phase of labor are usually allowed to walk.
   G. **Narcotic and analgesic drugs**
      1. Nalbuphine (Nubain) 5 to 10 mg SC or IV q2-3h.
      2. Butorphanol (Stadol) 2 mg IM q3-4h or 0.5-1.0 mg IV q1.5-2.0h **OR**
      3. Meperidine (Demerol) 50 to 100 mg IM q3-4h or 10 to 25 mg IV q1.5-3.0 h **OR**
      4. Narcotics should be avoided if their peak action will not have diminished by the time of delivery. Respiratory depression is reversed with naloxone (Narcan): Adults, 0.4 mg IV or IM and neonates, 0.01 mg/kg.
   H. **Epidural anesthesia**
      1. Contraindications include infection in the lumbar area, clotting defect, active neurologic disease, sensitivity to the anesthetic, hypovolemia, and septicemia.
      2. Risks include hypotension, respiratory arrest, toxic drug reaction, and rare neurologic complications. An epidural has no significant effect on the progress of labor.
      3. Before the epidural is initiated, the patient is hydrated with 500-1000 mL of dextrose-free intravenous fluid.

Labor and Delivery Admitting Orders

Admit: Labor and Delivery
Diagnoses: Intrauterine pregnancy at _____ weeks.
Condition: Satisfactory
Vitals: q1 hr per routine
Activity: May ambulate as tolerated.
Nursing: I and O. Catheterize prn; external or internal monitors.
Diet: NPO except ice chips.
IV Fluids: Lactated Ringers with 5% dextrose at 125 cc/h.
Medications:
Epidural at 4-5 cm.
Nalbuphine (Nubain) 5-10 mg IV/SC q2-3h prn **OR**
Butorphanol (Stadol) 0.5-1 mg IV q1.5-2h prn **OR**
Meperidine (Demerol) 25-75 mg slow IV q1.5-3h prn pain **AND**
Promethazine (Phenergan) 25-50 mg, IV q3-4h prn nausea **OR**
Hydroxyzine (Vistaril) 25-50 mg IV q3-4h prn
Fleet enema PR prn constipation.
Labs: CBC, dipstick urine protein, blood type and Rh, antibody screen,
VDRL, HBsAg, rubella, type and screen (C-section).

I. **Intrapartum antibiotic prophylaxis for group B streptococcus is recommended for the following:**
 1. Pregnant women with a positive screening culture unless a planned Cesarean section is performed in the absence of labor or rupture of membranes
 2. Pregnant women who gave birth to a previous infant with invasive GBS disease
 3. Pregnant women with documented GBS bacteriuria during the current pregnancy
 4. Pregnant women whose culture status is unknown (culture not performed or result not available) and who also have delivery at <37 weeks of gestation, amniotic membrane rupture for ≥18 hours, or intrapartum temperature ≥100.4°F (≥38°C)
 5. The recommended IAP regimen is penicillin G (5 million units IV initial dose, then 2.5 million units IV Q4h). In women with non-immediate-type penicillin-allergy, cefazolin (Ancef, 2 g initial dose, then 1 g Q8h) is recommended. Clindamycin (900 mg IV Q8h) or erythromycin (500 mg IV Q6h) are recommended for patients at high risk for anaphylaxis to penicillins as long as their GBS isolate is documented to be susceptible to both clindamycin and erythromycin.

IV. **Normal spontaneous vaginal delivery**
 A. **Preparation.** As the multiparous patient approaches complete dilatation or as the nulliparous patient begins to crown the fetal scalp, preparations are made for delivery.
 B. **Maternal position.** The mother is usually placed in the dorsal lithotomy position with left lateral tilt.
 C. **Delivery of a fetus in an occiput anterior position**
  1. **Delivery of the head**
   a. The fetal head is delivered by extension as the flexed head passes through the vaginal introitus.
   b. Once the fetal head has been delivered, external rotation to the occiput transverse position occurs.
   c. The oropharynx and nose of the fetus are suctioned with the bulb syringe. A finger is passed into the vagina along the fetal neck to check for a nuchal cord. If one is present, it is lifted over the vertex. If this cannot be accomplished, the cord is doubly clamped and divided.

    d. If shoulder dystocia is anticipated, the shoulders should be delivered immediately.

  2. Episiotomy consists of incision of the perineum, enlarging the vaginal orifice at the time of delivery. If indicated, an episiotomy should be performed when 3-4 cm of fetal scalp is visible.

    a. With adequate local or spinal anesthetic in place, a medial episiotomy is completed by incising the perineum toward the anus and into the vagina.

    b. Avoid cutting into the anal sphincter or the rectum. A short perineum may require a mediolateral episiotomy.

    c. Application of pressure at the perineal apex with a towel-covered hand helps to prevent extension of the episiotomy.

  3. Delivery of the anterior shoulder is accomplished by gentle downward traction on the fetal head. The posterior shoulder is delivered by upward traction.

  4. Delivery of the body. The infant is grasped around the back with the left hand, and the right hand is placed, near the vagina, under the baby's buttocks, supporting the infant's body. The infant's body is rotated toward the operator and supported by the operator's forearm, freeing the right hand to suction the mouth and nose. The baby's head should be kept lower than the body to facilitate drainage of secretions.

  5. Suctioning of the nose and oropharynx is repeated.

  6. The umbilical cord is doubly clamped and cut, leaving 2-3 cm of cord.

D. Delivery of the placenta

  1. The placenta usually separates spontaneously from the uterine wall within 5 minutes of delivery. Gentle fundal massage and gentle traction on the cord facilitates delivery of the placenta.

  2. The placenta should be examined for missing cotyledons or blind vessels. The cut end of the cord should be examined for 2 arteries and a vein. The absence of one umbilical artery suggests a congenital anomaly.

  3. Prophylaxis against excessive postpartum blood loss consists of external fundal massage and oxytocin (Pitocin), 20 units in 1000 mL of IV fluid at 100 drops/minute after delivery of the placenta. Oxytocin can cause marked hypotension if administered as a IV bolus.

  4. After delivery of the placenta, the birth canal is inspected for lacerations.

Delivery Note

1. Note the age, gravida, para, and gestational age.
2. Time of birth, type of birth (spontaneous vaginal delivery), position (left occiput anterior).
3. Bulb suctioned, sex, weight, APGAR scores, nuchal cord, and number of cord vessels.
4. Placenta expressed spontaneously intact. Describe episiotomy degree and repair technique.
5. Note lacerations of cervix, vagina, rectum, perineum.
6. Estimated blood loss:
7. Disposition: Mother to recovery room in stable condition. Infant to nursery in stable condition.

Routine Postpartum Orders

Transfer: To recovery room, then postpartum ward when stable.
Vitals: Check vitals, bleeding, fundus q15min x 1 hr or until stable, then q4h.
Activity: Ambulate in 2 hours if stable
Nursing Orders: If unable to void, straight catheterize; sitz baths prn with 1:1000 Betadine prn, ice pack to perineum prn, record urine output.
Diet: Regular
IV Fluids: D5LR at 125 cc/h. Discontinue when stable and taking PO diet.
Medications:
    Oxytocin (Pitocin) 20 units in 1 L D5LR at 100 drops/minute or 10 U IM.
    FeSO4 325 mg PO bid-tid.
Symptomatic Medications:
    Acetaminophen/codeine (Tylenol #3) 1-2 tab PO q3-4h prn **OR**
    Oxycodone/acetaminophen (Percocet) 1 tab q6h prn pain.
    Milk of magnesia 30 mL PO q6h prn constipation.
    Docusate Sodium (Colace) 100 mg PO bid.
    Dulcolax suppository PR prn constipation.
    A and D cream or Lanolin prn if breast feeding.
    Breast binder or tight brazier and ice packs prn if not to breast feed.
Labs: Hemoglobin/hematocrit in AM. Give rubella vaccine if titer <1:10.

Active Management of Labor

The active management of labor refers to active control over the course of labor. There are three essential elements to active management are careful diagnosis of labor by strict criteria, constant monitoring of labor, and prompt intervention (eg, amniotomy, high dose oxytocin) if progress is unsatisfactory.

I. **Criteria for active management of labor:**
   A. Nulliparous
   B. Term pregnancy
   C. Singleton infant in cephalic presentation
   D. No pregnancy complications
   E. Experiencing spontaneous onset of labor.
II. **Diagnosis of labor**
   A. The diagnosis of labor is made only when contractions are accompanied by any one of the following:
      1. Bloody show
      2. Rupture of the membranes
      3. Full cervical effacement
   B. Women who meet these criteria are admitted to the labor unit.
III. **Management of labor**
   A. **Rupture of membranes**. Intact fetal membranes are artificially ruptured one hour after the diagnosis of labor is made to permit assessment of the quantity of fluid and the presence of meconium. Rupture of the membranes may accelerate labor.

B. Progress during the first stage of labor

1. Satisfactory progress in the first stage of labor is confirmed by cervical dilatation of at least 1 cm per hour after the membranes have been ruptured.

2. In the absence of medical contraindications, labor that fails to progress at the foregoing rate is treated with oxytocin.

3. **Progress during the second stage of labor** is measured by fetal descent and rotation.

   a. The second stage of labor is divided into two phases: the first phase is the time from full dilatation until the fetal head reaches the pelvic floor; the second phase extends from the time the head reaches the pelvic floor to delivery of the infant.

   b. The first phase of the second stage is characterized by descent of the fetal head. If the fetal head is high in the pelvis at full dilatation, the woman often has no urge to push and should not be encouraged to do so. Oxytocin treatment may be useful if the fetal head fails to descend after a period of observation.

C. Administration of oxytocin. Oxytocin is administered for treatment of failure of labor to progress, unless its use is contraindicated. Oxytocin may only be administered if the following conditions are met:

1. Fetal membranes are ruptured
2. Absence of meconium in amniotic fluid
3. Singleton fetus in a vertex position
4. No evidence of fetal distress

High Dose Oxytocin (Pitocin) Regimen

Begin oxytocin 6 mU per minute IV
Increase dose by 6 mU per minute every 15 minutes
Maximum dose: 40 mU per minute

D. Failure to progress (dystocia) is diagnosed when the cervix fails to dilate at least 1 cm per hour during the first stage of labor or when the fetal head fails to descend during the second stage of labor. Three possible causes for failure to progress are possible (excluding malpresentations and hydrocephalus):

1. Inefficient uterine action
2. Occiput-posterior position
3. Cephalopelvic disproportion.

E. Inefficient uterine action is the most common cause of dystocia in the nulliparous gravida, especially early in labor. Secondary arrest of labor after previously satisfactory progress may be due to an occiput-posterior position or cephalopelvic disproportion. It is often difficult for the clinician to differentiate among these entities, thus oxytocin is administered in all cases of failure to progress (unless a contraindication exists).

F. In the first stage, progressive cervical dilatation of at least 1 cm per hour should occur within one hour of establishing efficient uterine contractions (five to seven contractions within 15 minutes) with oxytocin. The second stage is considered prolonged if it extends longer than two hours in women without epidural anesthesia and longer than three hours in women with epidural anesthesia despite adequate contractions and oxytocin augmentation.

References: See page 166.

Perineal Lacerations and Episiotomies

I. **First-degree laceration**
  A. A first degree perineal laceration extends only through the vaginal and perineal skin.
  B. **Repair:** Place a single layer of interrupted 3-O chromic or Vicryl sutures about 1 cm apart.

II. **Second-degree laceration and repair of midline episiotomy**
  A. A second degree laceration extends deeply into the soft tissues of the perineum, down to, but not including, the external anal sphincter capsule. The disruption involves the bulbocavernosus and transverse perineal muscles.
  B. **Repair**
    1. Proximate the deep tissues of the perineal body by placing 3-4 interrupted 2-O or 3-O chromic or Vicryl absorbable sutures. Reapproximate the superficial layers of the perineal body with a running suture extending to the bottom of the episiotomy.
    2. Identify the apex of the vaginal laceration. Suture the vaginal mucosa with running, interlocking, 3-O chromic or Vicryl absorbable suture.
    3. Close the perineal skin with a running, subcuticular suture. Tie off the suture and remove the needle.

III. **Third-degree laceration**
  A. This laceration extends through the perineum and through the anal sphincter.
  B. **Repair**
    1. Identify each severed end of the external anal sphincter capsule, and grasp each end with an Allis clamp.
    2. Proximate the capsule of the sphincter with 4 interrupted sutures of 2-O or 3-O Vicryl suture, making sure the sutures do not penetrate the rectal mucosa.
    3. Continue the repair as for a second degree laceration as above. Stool softeners and sitz baths are prescribed post-partum.

IV. **Fourth-degree laceration**
  A. The laceration extends through the perineum, anal sphincter, and extends through the rectal mucosa to expose the lumen of the rectum.
  B. **Repair**
    1. Irrigate the laceration with sterile saline solution. Identify the anatomy, including the apex of the rectal mucosal laceration.
    2. Approximate the rectal submucosa with a running suture using a 3-O chromic on a GI needle extending to the margin of the anal skin.
    3. Place a second layer of running suture to invert the first suture line, and take some tension from the first layer closure.
    4. Identify and grasp the torn edges of the external anal sphincter capsule with Allis clamps, and perform a repair as for a third-degree laceration. Close the remaining layers as for a second-degree laceration.
    5. A low-residue diet, stool softeners, and sitz baths are prescribed post-partum.

References: See page 166.

Fetal Heart Rate Assessment

Fetal heart rate (FHR) assessment evaluates the fetal condition by identifying FHR patterns that may be associated with adverse fetal or neonatal outcome or are reassuring of fetal well-being.

I. **Fetal monitoring techniques**
  A. **Electronic fetal monitoring.** The electronic fetal monitor determines the FHR and continuously records it in graphical form.

B. **External fetal monitoring.** The FHR is measured by focusing an ultrasound beam on the fetal heart. The fetal monitor interprets Doppler signals.

C. **Internal fetal monitoring** of FHR is an invasive procedure. A spiral electrode is inserted transcervically into the fetal scalp. The internal electrode detects the fetal (ECG) and calculates the fetal heart rate based upon the interval between R waves. This signal provides accurate measurement of beat-to-beat and baseline variability.

D. **Biophysical profile.** The biophysical profile (BPP) consists of electronic fetal heart rate evaluation combined with sonographically assessed fetal breathing movements, motor movement, gross fetal tone, and amniotic fluid volume.

II. **Fetal heart rate patterns**

A. The fetal heart rate pattern recorded by an electronic fetal monitor is categorized as reassuring or nonreassuring.

B. **Reassuring fetal heart rate patterns**
   1. A baseline fetal heart rate of 120 to 160 bpm
   2. Absence of FHR decelerations
   3. Age appropriate FHR accelerations
   4. Normal FHR variability (5 to 25 bpm).

C. **Early decelerations** (ie, shallow symmetrical decelerations in which the nadir of the deceleration occurs simultaneously with the peak of the contraction) and mild bradycardia of 100 to 119 bpm are caused by fetal head compression, and they are not associated with fetal acidosis or poor neonatal outcome.

D. The majority of fetal arrhythmias are benign and spontaneously convert to normal sinus rhythm by 24 hours after birth. Persistent tachyarrhythmias may cause fetal hydrops if present for many hours to days. Persistent bradyarrhythmias are often associated with fetal heart disease (eg, cardiomyopathy related to lupus), but seldom result in hypoxia or acidosis in fetal life.

E. FHR accelerations and mild variable decelerations are indicative of a normally functioning autonomic nervous system.

F. **Nonreassuring fetal heart rate patterns**
   1. Nonreassuring FHR patterns are nonspecific and require further evaluation. The fetus may not be acidotic initially; however, continuation or worsening of the clinical situation may result in fetal acidosis.
   2. **Late decelerations** are characterized by a smooth U-shaped fall in the fetal heart rate beginning after the contraction has started and ending after the contraction has ended. The nadir of the deceleration occurs after the peak of the contraction. Mild late decelerations are a reflex central nervous system response to hypoxia, while severe late decelerations suggest direct myocardial depression.
   3. **Sinusoidal heart rate** is defined as a pattern of regular variability resembling a sine wave with a fixed periodicity of three to five cycles per minute and an amplitude of 5 to 40 bpm. The sinusoidal pattern is caused by moderate fetal hypoxemia, often secondary to fetal anemia.
   4. **Variable decelerations** are characterized by the variable onset of abrupt slowing of the FHR in association with uterine contractions. Mild or moderate variable decelerations do not have a late component, are of short duration and depth, and end by rapid return to a normal baseline FHR. They are usually intermittent. This pattern is not associated with acidosis or low Apgar scores. Severe variable decelerations have a late component during which the fetal pH falls. They also may display loss of variability or rebound tachycardia and last longer than 60 seconds or fall to less than 70 bpm. They tend to become persistent and progressively deeper and longer lasting over time.
   5. **Fetal distress patterns**
      a. Fetal distress is likely to cause fetal or neonatal death or damage if left uncorrected. Fetal distress patterns are associated with fetal acidemia and hypoxemia.

      b. Undulating baseline. Alternating tachycardia and bradycardia, often with reduced variability between the wide swings in heart rate.

      c. Severe bradycardia. Fetal heart rate below 100 bpm for a prolonged period of time (ie, at least 10 minutes).

      d. Tachycardia with diminished variability that is unrelated to drugs or additional non-reassuring periodic patterns (eg, late decelerations or severe variable decelerations)

III. Intrapartum fetal surveillance

A. Transient episodes of hypoxemia and hypoxia are generally well-tolerated by the fetus. Progressive or severe episodes may lead to fetal acidosis and subsequent asphyxia. One goal of intrapartum fetal surveillance is to distinguish the fetus with FHR abnormalities who is well compensated from one who is at risk for neurological impairment or death. Ancillary tests are useful for this purpose.

B. Ancillary tests

    1. Fetal scalp stimulation. Fetal scalp stimulation is similar to the vibroacoustic stimulation test used antepartum. Absence of acidosis (ie, fetal pH greater than 7.20) is confirmed by elicitation of a FHR acceleration when an examiner stimulates the fetal vertex with the examining finger. Fetal scalp sampling is recommended to further evaluate positive test results.

    2. Fetal scalp blood sampling. Capillary blood collected from the fetal scalp typically has a pH lower than arterial blood. A pH of 7.20 was initially thought to represent the critical value for identifying serious fetal stress and an increase in the incidence of low Apgar scores. The degree of technical skill required prohibits widespread use of this modality.

IV. Management of nonreassuring FHR patterns during labor

    1. Determine the cause of the abnormality (eg, cord prolapse, maternal medication, abruption placenta)

    2. Attempt to correct the problem or initiate measures to improve fetal oxygenation (eg, change maternal position, administer oxygen and intravenous fluids, consider amnioinfusion or tocolysis)

    3. If the nonreassuring pattern does not resolve within a few minutes, perform ancillary tests to determine the fetal condition

    4. Determine whether operative intervention is needed

B. The presence of accelerations almost always assures the absence of fetal acidosis. Therefore, if such accelerations are not observed, they should be elicited by manual or vibroacoustic stimulation. There is a 50 percent risk of fetal acidosis in fetuses in whom accelerations cannot be elicited, so further evaluation by fetal scalp sampling for pH is indicated to help clarify the fetal acid-base status. Serial evaluation every 20 to 30 minutes is necessary if the FHR pattern remains nonreassuring. Expeditious delivery is indicated for persistent nonreassuring FHR patterns.

Management of Variant Fetal Heart Rate Patterns		
FHR Pattern	**Diagnosis**	**Action**
Normal rate normal variability, accelerations, no decelerations	Fetus is well oxygenated	None
Normal variability, accelerations, mild nonreassuring pattern (bradycardia, late decelerations, variable decelerations)	Fetus is still well oxygenated centrally	Conservative management.

FHR Pattern	Diagnosis	Action
Normal variability, ± accelerations, moderate-severe nonreassuring pattern (bradycardia, late decelerations, variable decelerations)	Fetus is still well oxygenated centrally, but the FHR suggests hypoxia	Continue conservative management. Consider stimulation testing. Prepare for rapid delivery if pattern worsens
Decreasing variability, ± accelerations, moderate-severe nonreassuring patterns (bradycardia, late decelerations, variable decelerations)	Fetus may be on the verge of decompensation	Deliver if spontaneous delivery is remote, or if stimulation supports diagnosis of decompensation. Normal response to stimulation may allow time to await a vaginal delivery
Absent variability, no accelerations, moderate/severe nonreassuring patterns (bradycardia, late decelerations, variable decelerations)	Evidence of actual or impending asphyxia	Deliver. Stimulation or in-utero management may be attempted if delivery is not delayed

References: See page 166.

Antepartum Fetal Surveillance

I. **Antepartum fetal surveillance techniques**
   A. Antepartum fetal surveillance should be initiated in pregnancies in which the risk of fetal demise is known to be increased. These problems can include maternal conditions such as antiphospholipid syndrome, chronic hypertension, renal disease, systemic lupus erythematosus, or type 1 diabetes mellitus. Monitoring should also be initiated in pregnancy-related conditions such as preeclampsia, intrauterine growth restriction (IUGR), multiple gestation, poor obstetrical history, or postterm pregnancy.
   B. Antepartum fetal surveillance can include the nonstress test (NST), BPP, oxytocin challenge test (OCT), or modified BPP.
   C. **Nonstress test**
      1. A NST is performed using an electronic fetal monitor. Testing is generally begun at 32 to 34 weeks. Testing is performed at daily to weekly intervals as long as the indication for testing persists.
      2. The test is reactive if there are two or more fetal heart rate accelerations of 15 bpm above the baseline rate lasting for 15 seconds in a 20 minute period. A nonreactive NST does not show such accelerations over a 40 minute period. Nonreactivity may be related to fetal immaturity, a sleep cycle, drugs, fetal anomalies, or fetal hypoxemia.
      3. If the NST is nonreactive, it is considered nonreassuring and further evaluation or delivery of the fetus is indicated. At term, delivery rather than further evaluation is usually warranted. A nonreassuring NST preterm usually should be assessed with ancillary tests, since the false positive rate of an isolated NST may be 50 to 60 percent.
   D. **Fetal movement assessment ("kick counts")**
      1. A diminution in the maternal perception of fetal movement often but not invariably precedes fetal death, in some cases by several days.
      2. The woman lies on her side and counts distinct fetal movements. Perception of 10 distinct movements in a period of up to 2 hours is considered reassuring. Once 10 movements have been perceived, the count may be discontinued. In the absence of a reassuring count, non stress testing is recommended.

Indications for Antepartum Fetal Surveillance	
Maternal	**Pregnancy complications**
antiphospholipid syndrome	preeclampsia
poorly controlled hyperthyroidism	decreased fetal movement
hemoglobinopathies	oligohydramnios
cyanotic heart disease	polyhydramnios
systemic lupus erythematosus	Intrauterine growth restriction
chronic renal disease	postterm pregnancy
type I diabetes mellitus	isoimmunization
hypertensive disorders	previous unexplained fetal demise
	multiple gestation

E. Ancillary tests
   1. **Vibroacoustic stimulation** is performed by placing an artificial larynx on the maternal abdomen and delivering a short burst of sound to the fetus. The procedure can shorten the duration of time needed to produce reactivity and the frequency of nonreactive NSTs, without compromising the predictive value of a reactive NST.
   2. **Oxytocin challenge test**
      a. The oxytocin challenge test (OCT) is done by intravenously infusing dilute oxytocin until three contractions occur within ten minutes. The test is interpreted as follows:
      b. A positive test is defined by the presence of late decelerations following 50 percent or more of the contractions
      c. A negative test has no late or significant variable decelerations
      d. An equivocal-suspicious pattern consists of intermittent late or significant variable decelerations, while an equivocal-hyperstimulatory pattern refers to fetal heart rate decelerations occurring with contractions more frequent than every two minutes or lasting longer than 90 seconds
      e. An unsatisfactory test is one in which the tracing is uninterpretable or contractions are fewer than three in 10 minutes
      f. A positive test indicates decreased fetal reserve and correlates with a 20 to 40 percent incidence of abnormal FHR patterns during labor. An equivocal-suspicious test with repetitive variable decelerations is also associated with abnormal FHR patterns in labor, which are often related to cord compression due to oligohydramnios.
   3. **Fetal biophysical profile**
      a. The fetal biophysical profile score refers to the sonographic assessment of four biophysical variables: fetal movement, fetal tone, fetal breathing, amniotic fluid volume and nonstress testing. Each of these five parameters is given a score of 0 or 2 points, depending upon whether specific criteria are met. Fetal BPS is a noninvasive, highly accurate means for predicting the presence of fetal asphyxia.
      b. **Criteria**
         (1) A normal variable is assigned a score of two and an abnormal variable a score of zero. The maximal score is 10/10 and the minimal score is 0/10.
         (2) **Amniotic fluid volume** is based upon an ultrasound-based objective measurement of the largest visible pocket. The selected largest pocket must have a transverse diameter of at least one centimeter.

Components of the Biophysical Profile		
Parameter	**Normal (score = 2)**	**Abnormal (score = 0)**
Nonstress test	≥2 accelerations ≥15 beats per minute above baseline during test lasting ≥15 seconds in 20 minutes	<2 accelerations
Amniotic fluid volume	Amniotic fluid index >5 or at least 1 pocket measuring 2 cm x 2 cm in perpendicular planes	AFI <5 or no pocket >2 cm x 2 cm
Fetal breathing movement	Sustained FBM (≥30 seconds)	Absence of FBM or short gasps only <30 seconds total
Fetal body movements	≥3 episodes of either limb or trunk movement	<3 episodes during test
Fetal tone	Extremities in flexion at rest and ≥1 episode of extension of extremity, hand or spine with return to flexion	Extension at rest or no return to flexion after movement

A total score of 8 to 10 is reassuring; a score of 6 is suspicious, and a score of 4 or less is ominous.
Amniotic fluid index = the sum of the largest vertical pocket in each of four quadrants on the maternal abdomen intersecting at the umbilicus.

- c. **Clinical utility**
  - (1) The fetal BPS is noninvasive and highly accurate for predicting the presence of fetal asphyxia. The probability of fetal acidemia is virtually zero when the score is normal (8 to 10). The false negative rate (ie, fetal death within one week of a last test with a normal score) is exceedingly low. The likelihood of fetal compromise and death rises as the score falls.
  - (2) The risk of fetal demise within one week of a normal test result is 0.8 per 1000 women tested. The positive predictive value of the BPS for evidence of true fetal compromise is only 50 percent, with a negative predictive value greater than 99.9 percent.
- d. **Indications and frequency of testing**
  - (1) ACOG recommends antepartum testing in the following situations:
    - (a) Women with high-risk factors for fetal asphyxia should undergo antepartum fetal surveillance with tests (eg, BPS, nonstress test)
    - (b) Testing may be initiated as early as 26 weeks of gestation when clinical conditions suggest early fetal compromise is likely. Initiating testing at 32 to 34 weeks of gestation is appropriate for most pregnancies at increased risk of stillbirth.
    - (c) A reassuring test (eg, BPS of 8 to 10) should be repeated periodically (weekly or twice weekly) until delivery when the high-risk condition persists.
    - (d) Any significant deterioration in the clinical status (eg, worsening preeclampsia, decreased fetal activity) requires fetal reevaluation.

       (e) Severe oligohydramnios (no vertical pocket >2 cm or amniotic fluid index ≤5) requires either delivery or close maternal and fetal surveillance.

       (f) Induction of labor may be attempted with abnormal antepartum testing as long as the fetal heart rate and contractions are monitored continuously and are reassuring. Cesarean delivery is indicated if there are repetitive late decelerations.

(2) The minimum gestational age for testing should reflect the lower limit that intervention with delivery would be considered. This age is now 24 to 25 weeks.

(3) Modified biophysical profile. Assessment of amniotic fluid volume and nonstress testing appear to be as reliable a predictor of long-term fetal well-being as the full BPS. The rate of stillbirth within one week of a normal modified BPS is the same as with the full BPS, 0.8 per 1000 women tested.

Guidelines for Antepartum Testing

Indication	Initiation	Frequency
Post-term pregnancy	41 weeks	Twice a week
Preterm rupture of membranes	At onset	Daily
Bleeding	26 weeks or at onset	Twice a week
Oligohydramnios	26 weeks or at onset	Twice a week
Polyhydramnios	32 weeks	Weekly
Diabetes	32 weeks	Twice a week
Chronic or pregnancy-induced hypertension	28 weeks	Weekly. Increase to twice-weekly at 32 weeks.
Steroid-dependent or poorly controlled asthma	28 weeks	Weekly
Sickle cell disease	32 weeks (earlier if symptoms)	Weekly (more often if severe)
Impaired renal function	28 weeks	Weekly
Substance abuse	32 weeks	Weekly
Prior stillbirth	At 2 weeks before prior fetal death	Weekly
Multiple gestation	32 weeks	Weekly
Congenital anomaly	32 weeks	Weekly
Fetal growth restriction	26 weeks	Twice a week or at onset
Decreased fetal movement	At time of complaint	Once

F. **Perinatal outcome.** An abnormal NST result should be interpreted with caution. Further assessment of fetal condition using the NST, OCT, or BPP should usually be performed to help determine whether the fetus is in immediate jeopardy.

G. **Management of abnormal test results**

1. Maternal reports of decreased fetal movement should be evaluated by an NST, CST, BPP, or modified BPP. These results, if normal, usually are sufficient to exclude imminent fetal jeopardy. A nonreactive NST or an abnormal modified BPP generally should be followed by additional testing (either a CST or a full BPP). In many circumstances, a positive CST result generally indicates that delivery is warranted.

2. A BPP score of 6 is considered equivocal; in the term fetus, this score generally should prompt delivery, whereas in the preterm fetus, it should result in a repeat BPP in 24 hours. In the interim, maternal corticosteroid administration should be considered for pregnancies of less than 34 weeks of gestation. Repeat equivocal scores should result either in delivery or continued intensive surveillance. A BPP score of 4 usually indicates that delivery is warranted.

3. Preterm delivery is indicated for nonreassuring antepartum fetal testing results that have been confirmed by additional testing. At term, additional testing can be omitted since the risk from delivery is small. Depending on the fetal heart rate pattern, induction of labor with continuous FHR and contraction monitoring may be attempted in the absence of obstetrical contraindications. Repetitive late decelerations or severe variable decelerations usually require cesarean delivery.

References: See page 166.

Brief Postoperative Cesarean Section Note

Pre-op diagnosis:
1. 23 year old G_1P_0, estimated gestational age = 40 weeks
2. Dystocia
3. Non-reassuring fetal tracing

Post-op diagnosis: Same as above
Procedure: Primary low segment transverse cesarean section
Attending Surgeon, Assistant:
Anesthesia: Epidural
Operative Findings: Weight and sex of infant, APGARs at 1 min and 5 min; normal uterus, tubes, ovaries.
Cord pH:
Specimens: Placenta, cord blood (type and Rh).
Estimated Blood Loss: 800 cc; no blood replaced.
Fluids, blood and urine output:
Drains: Foley to gravity.
Complications: None
Disposition: Patient sent to recovery room in stable condition.

Cesarean Section Operative Report

Preoperative Diagnosis:
1. 23 year old G_1P_0, estimated gestational age = 40 weeks
2. Dystocia
3. Non-reassuring fetal tracing

Postoperative Diagnosis: Same as above
Title of Operation: Primary low segment transverse cesarean section
Surgeon:
Assistant:
Anesthesia: Epidural
Findings At Surgery: Male infant in occiput posterior presentation. Thin meconium with none below the cords, pediatrics present at delivery, APGAR's 6/8, weight 3980 g. Normal uterus, tubes, and ovaries.

Description of Operative Procedure:

After assuring informed consent, the patient was taken to the operating room and spinal anesthesia was initiated. The patient was placed in the dorsal, supine position with left lateral tilt. The abdomen was prepped and draped in sterile fashion.

A Pfannenstiel skin incision was made with a scalpel and carried through to the level of the fascia. The fascial incision was extended bilaterally with Mayo scissors. The fascial incision was then grasped with the Kocher clamps, elevated, and sharply and bluntly dissected superiorly and inferiorly from the rectus muscles.

The rectus muscles were then separated in the midline, and the peritoneum was tented up, and entered sharply with Metzenbaum scissors. The peritoneal incision was extended superiorly and inferiorly with good visualization of the bladder.

A bladder blade was then inserted, and the vesicouterine peritoneum was identified, grasped with the pick-ups, and entered sharply with the Metzenbaum scissors. This incision was then extended laterally, and a bladder flap was created. The bladder was retracted using the bladder blade. The lower uterine segment was incised in a transverse fashion with the scalpel, then extended bilaterally with bandage scissors. The bladder blade was removed, and the infants head was delivered atraumatically. The nose and mouth were suctioned and the cord clamped and cut. The infant was handed off to the pediatrician. Cord gases and cord blood were sent.

The placenta was then removed manually, and the uterus was exteriorized, and cleared of all clots and debris. The uterine incision was repaired with 1-O chromic in a running locking fashion. A second layer of 1-O chromic was used to obtain excellent hemostasis. The bladder flap was repaired with a 3-O Vicryl in a running fashion. The cul-de-sac was cleared of clots and the uterus was returned to the abdomen. The peritoneum was closed with 3-0 Vicryl. The fascia was reapproximated with O Vicryl in a running fashion. The skin was closed with staples.

The patient tolerated the procedure well. Needle and sponge counts were correct times two. Two grams of Ancef was given at cord clamp, and a sterile dressing was placed over the incision.

Estimated Blood Loss (EBL): 800 cc; no blood replaced (normal blood loss is 500-1000 cc).
Specimens: Placenta, cord pH, cord blood specimens.
Drains: Foley to gravity.
Fluids: Input - 2000 cc LR; Output - 300 cc clear urine.
Complications: None.
Disposition: The patient was taken to the recovery room then postpartum ward in stable condition.

Postoperative Management after Cesarean Section

I. Post Cesarean Section Orders
  A. **Transfer:** to post partum ward when stable.
  B. **Vital signs:** q4h x 24 hours, I and O.
  C. **Activity:** Bed rest x 6-8 hours, then ambulate; if given spinal, keep patient flat on back x 8h. Incentive spirometer q1h while awake.
  D. **Diet:** NPO x 8h, then sips of water. Advance to clear liquids, then to regular diet as tolerated.
  E. **IV Fluids:** IV D5 LR or D5 ½ NS at 125 cc/h. Foley to gravity; discontinue after 12 hours. I and O catheterize prn.
  F. **Medications**
    1. Cefazolin (Ancef) 1 gm IVPB x one dose at time of cesarean section.
    2. Nalbuphine (Nubain) 5 to 10 mg SC or IV q2-3h **OR**
    3. Meperidine (Demerol) 50-75 mg IM q3-4h prn pain.
    4. Hydroxyzine (Vistaril) 25-50 mg IM q3-4h prn nausea.
    5. Prochlorperazine (Compazine) 10 mg IV q4-6h prn nausea **OR**
    6. Promethazine (Phenergan) 25-50 mg IV q3-4h prn nausea
  G. **Labs:** CBC in AM.

II. Postoperative Day #1
  A. Assess pain, lungs, cardiac status, fundal height, lochia, passing of flatus, bowel movement, distension, tenderness, bowel sounds, incision.
  B. Discontinue IV when taking adequate PO fluids.
  C. Discontinue Foley, and I and O catheterize prn.
  D. Ambulate tid with assistance; incentive spirometer q1h while awake.
  E. Check hematocrit, hemoglobin, Rh, and rubella status.
  F. **Medications**
    1. Acetaminophen/codeine (Tylenol #3) 1-2 PO q4-6h prn pain **OR**
    2. Oxycodone/acetaminophen (Percocet) 1 tab q6h prn pain.
    3. FeSO4 325 mg PO bid-tid.
    4. Multivitamin PO qd, Colace 100 mg PO bid. Mylicon 80 mg PO qid prn bloating.

III. Postoperative Day #2
  A. If passing gas and/or bowel movement, advance to regular diet.
  B. Laxatives: Dulcolax supp prn or Milk of magnesia 30 cc PO tid prn. Mylicon 80 mg PO qid prn bloating.

IV. Postoperative Day #3
  A. If transverse incision, remove staples and place steri-strips on day 3. If a vertical incision, remove staples on post op day 5.
  B. Discharge home on appropriate medications; follow up in 2 and 6 weeks.

Laparoscopic Bilateral Tubal Ligation Operative Report

Preoperative Diagnosis: Multiparous female desiring permanent sterilization.
Postoperative Diagnosis: Same as above
Title of Operation: Laparoscopic bilateral tubal ligation with Falope rings
Surgeon:
Assistant:
Anesthesia: General endotracheal
Findings At Surgery: Normal uterus, tubes, and ovaries.
Description of Operative Procedure

After informed consent, the patient was taken to the operating room where general anesthesia was administered. The patient was examined under anesthesia and found to have a normal uterus with normal adnexa. She was placed in the dorsal lithotomy position and prepped and draped in sterile fashion. A bivalve speculum was placed in the vagina, and the anterior lip of the cervix was grasped with a single toothed tenaculum. A uterine manipulator was placed into the endocervical canal and articulated with the tenaculum. The speculum was removed from the vagina.

An infraumbilical incision was made with a scalpel, then while tenting up on the abdomen, a Verres needle was admitted into the intraabdominal cavity. A saline drop test was performed and noted to be within normal limits. Pneumoperitoneum was attained with 4 liters of carbon dioxide. The Verres needle was removed, and a 10 mm trocar and sleeve were advanced into the intraabdominal cavity while tenting up on the abdomen. The laparoscope was inserted and proper location was confirmed. A second incision was made 2 cm above the symphysis pubis, and a 5 mm trocar and sleeve were inserted into the abdomen under laparoscopic visualization without complication.

A survey revealed normal pelvic and abdominal anatomy. A Falope ring applicator was advanced through the second trocar sleeve, and the left Fallopian tube was identified. The tube was followed out to the fimbriated end, and grasped 4 cm from the cornual region. The Falope ring was applied to a knuckle of tube and good blanching was noted at the site of application. No bleeding was observed from the mesosalpinx. The Falope ring applicator was reloaded, and a Falope ring was applied in a similar fashion to the opposite tube. Carbon dioxide was allowed to escape from the abdomen.

The instruments were removed, and the skin incisions were closed with #3-O Vicryl in a subcuticular fashion. The instruments were removed from the vagina, and excellent hemostasis was noted. The patient tolerated the procedure well, and sponge, lap and needle counts were correct times two. The patient was taken to the recovery room in stable condition.

Estimated Blood Loss (EBL): <10 cc
Specimens: None
Drains: Foley to gravity
Fluids: 1500 cc LR
Complications: None
Disposition: The patient was taken to the recovery room in stable condition.

Postpartum Tubal Ligation Operative Report

Preoperative Diagnosis: Multiparous female after vaginal delivery, desiring permanent sterilization.
Postoperative Diagnosis: Same as above
Title of Operation: Modified Pomeroy bilateral tubal ligation
Surgeon:
Assistant:
Anesthesia: Epidural
Findings At Surgery: Normal fallopian tubes bilaterally
Description of Operative Procedure:

After assuring informed consent, the patient was taken to the operating room and spinal anesthesia administered. A small, transverse, infraumbilical skin incision was made with a scalpel, and the incision was carried down through the underlying fascia until the peritoneum was identified and entered. The left fallopian tube was identified, brought into the incision and grasped with a Babcock clamp. The tube was then followed out to the fimbria. An avascular midsection of the fallopian tube was grasped with a Babcock clamp and brought into a knuckle. The tube was doubly ligated with an O-plain suture and transected. The specimen was sent to pathology. Excellent hemostasis was noted, and the tube was returned to the abdomen. The same procedure was performed on the opposite fallopian tube.

The fascia was then closed with O-Vicryl in a single layer. The skin was closed with 3-O Vicryl in a subcuticular fashion. The patient tolerated the procedure well. Needle and sponge counts were correct times 2.

Estimated Blood Loss (EBL): <20 cc
Specimens: Segments of right and left tubes
Drains: Foley to gravity
Fluids: Input - 500 cc LR; output - 300 cc clear urine

Complications: None
Disposition: The patient was taken to the recovery room in stable condition.

Prevention of D Isoimmunization

The morbidity and mortality of Rh hemolytic disease can be significantly reduced by identification of women at risk for isoimmunization and by administration of D immunoglobulin. Administration of D immunoglobulin [RhoGAM, Rho(D) immunoglobulin, RhIg] is very effective in the preventing isoimmunization to the D antigen.

I. **Prenatal testing**
   A. Routine prenatal laboratory evaluation includes ABO and D blood type determination and antibody screen.
   B. At 28-29 weeks of gestation woman who are D negative but not D isoimmunized should be retested for D antibody. If the test reveals that no D antibody is present, prophylactic D immunoglobulin [RhoGAM, Rho(D) immunoglobulin, RhIg] is indicated.
   C. If D antibody is present, D immunoglobulin will not be beneficial, and specialized management of the D isoimmunized pregnancy is undertaken to manage hemolytic disease of the fetus and hydrops fetalis.

II. **Routine administration of D immunoglobulin**
   A. **Abortion.** D sensitization may be caused by abortion. D sensitization occurs more frequently after induced abortion than after spontaneous abortion, and it occurs more frequently after late abortion than after early abortion. D sensitization occurs following induced abortion in 4-5% of susceptible women. All unsensitized, D-negative women who have an induced or spontaneous abortion should be treated with D immunoglobulin unless the father is known to be D negative.
   B. **Dosage** of D immunoglobulin is determined by the stage of gestation. If the abortion occurs before 13 weeks of gestation, 50 mcg of D immunoglobulin prevents sensitization. For abortions occurring at 13 weeks of gestation and later, 300-mcg is given.
   C. **Ectopic pregnancy** can cause D sensitization. All unsensitized, D-negative women who have an ectopic pregnancy should be given D immunoglobulin. The dosage is determined by the gestational age, as described above for abortion.
   D. **Amniocentesis**
      1. D isoimmunization can occur after amniocentesis. D immunoglobulin, 300 mcg, should be administered to unsensitized, D-negative, susceptible patients following first- and second-trimester amniocentesis.
      2. Following third-trimester amniocentesis, 300 mcg of D immunoglobulin should be administered. If amniocentesis is performed and delivery is planned within 48 hours, D immunoglobulin can be withheld until after delivery, when the newborn can be tested for D positivity. If the amniocentesis is expected to precede delivery by more than 48 hours, the patient should receive 300 mcg of D immunoglobulin at the time of amniocentesis.
   E. **Antepartum prophylaxis**
      1. Isoimmunized occurs in 1-2% of D-negative women during the antepartum period. D immunoglobulin, administered both during pregnancy and postpartum, can reduce the incidence of D isoimmunization to 0.3%.
      2. Antepartum prophylaxis is given at 28-29 weeks of gestation. Antibody-negative, Rh-negative gravidas should have a repeat assessment at 28 weeks of gestation. D immunoglobulin (RhoGAM, RhIg), 300 mcg, is given to D-negative women. However, if the father of the fetus is known with certainty to be D negative, antepartum prophylaxis is not necessary.

F. Postpartum D immunoglobulin
1. D immunoglobulin is given to the D negative mother as soon after delivery as cord blood findings indicate that the baby is Rh positive.
2. A woman at risk who is inadvertently not given D immunoglobulin within 72 hours after delivery should still receive prophylaxis at any time up until two weeks after delivery. If prophylaxis is delayed, it may not be effective.
3. A quantitative Kleihauer-Betke analysis should be performed in situations in which significant maternal bleeding may have occurred (eg, after maternal abdominal trauma, abruptio placentae, external cephalic version). If the quantitative determination is thought to be more than 30 mL, D immune globulin should be given to the mother in multiples of one vial (300 mcg) for each 30 mL of estimated fetal whole blood in her circulation, unless the father of the baby is known to be D negative.

G. Abruptio placentae, placenta previa, cesarean delivery, intrauterine manipulation, or manual removal of the placenta may cause more than 30 mL of fetal-to-maternal bleeding. In these conditions, testing for excessive bleeding (Kleihauer-Betke test) or inadequate D immunoglobulin dosage (indirect Coombs test) is necessary.

References: See page 166.

Complications of Pregnancy

Nausea and Vomiting of Pregnancy and Hyperemesis Gravidarum

Nausea and vomiting to affects about 70% to 85% of pregnant women. Symptoms of nausea and vomiting of pregnancy (NVP) are most common during the first trimester; however, some women have persistent nausea for their entire pregnancy. Hyperemesis often occurs in association with high levels of human chorionic gonadotropin (hCG), such as with multiple pregnancies, trophoblastic disease, and fetal anomalies such as triploidy.

Conditions that Predispose to Excessive Nausea and Vomiting
Viral gastroenteritis
Gestational trophoblastic disease
Hepatitis
Urinary tract infection
Multifetal gestation
Gallbladder disease
Migraine

I. **Treatment of nausea and vomiting of pregnancy**
   A. Patients should avoid odors or foods that seem to be aggravating the nausea. Useful dietary modifications include avoiding fatty or spicy foods, and stopping iron supplements. Frequent small meals also may improve symptoms. Recommendations include bland and dry foods, high-protein snacks, and crackers at the bedside to be taken first thing in the morning.
   B. Cholecystitis, peptic ulcer disease, or hepatitis can cause nausea and vomiting and should be excluded. Gastroenteritis, appendicitis, pyelonephritis, and pancreatitis also should be excluded. Obstetric explanations for nausea and vomiting may include multiple pregnancies or a hydatidiform mole.
   C. Non-pharmacologic remedies are adequate for up to 90% of patients with NVP. However, about 10% will require medication and about 1% have severe enough vomiting that they require hospitalization.
   D. **Vitamin therapy.** Pyridoxine is effective as first-line therapy and is recommended up to 25 mg three times daily. Pyridoxine serum levels do not appear to correlate with the prevalence or degree of nausea and vomiting. Multivitamins also are effective for prevention of NVP. Premesis Rx is a prescription tablet with controlled-release vitamin B6, 75 mg, so it can be given once a day. It also contains vitamin B12 (12 mcg), folic acid (1 mg), and calcium carbonate (200 mg).
   E. **Over-the-Counter Therapy.** If pyridoxine alone is not efficacious, an alternative is to combine over-the-counter doxylamine 25 mg (Unisom) and pyridoxine 25 mg. One could combine the 25 mg of pyridoxine three times daily with doxylamine 25 mg, 1 tablet every bedtime, and ½ tablet morning and afternoon. There is no evidence that doxylamine is a teratogen.

Drug Therapy for Nausea and Vomiting of Pregnancy	
Generic name (trade name)	**Dosage**
Antihistamines	
Doxylamine (Unisom)	25 mg ½ tab BID, 1 tab qhs
Dimenhydrinate (Dramamine)	25 to 100 mg po/im/iv every 4 to 6 hr
Diphenhydramine (Benadryl)	25 to 50 mg po/im/iv every 4 to 6 hr
Trimethobenzamide (Tigan)	250 mg po every 6 to 8 hr or 200 mg im/pr every 6 to 8 hr
Meclizine (Antivert)	12.5 to 25 mg BID/TID
Phenothiazines	
Promethazine (Phenergan)	12.5 to 25 mg po/iv/pr every 4 to 6 hr
Prochlorperazine (Compazine)	5 to 10 mg po/iv every 6 to 8 hr or 25 mg pr every 6 to 8 hr
Prokinetic agents	
Metoclopramide (Reglan)	10 to 20 mg po/iv every 6 hr
Serotonin (5-HT$_3$) antagonists	
Ondansetron (Zofran)	8 mg po/iv every 8 hr
Corticosteroids	
Methylprednisolone (Medrol)	16 mg po TID for 3 days then ½ dose every 3 days for 2 wks

F. **Pharmacologic Therapy**
   1. Prescribed medication is the next step if dietary modifications and vitamin B6 therapy with doxylamine are ineffective. The phenothiazines are safe and effective, and promethazine (Phenergan) often is tried first. One of the disadvantages of the phenothiazines is their potential for dystonic effects.
   2. **Metoclopramide (Reglan)** is the antiemetic drug of choice in pregnancy in several European countries. There was no increased risk of birth defects.
   3. **Ondansetron (Zofran)** has been compared with promethazine (Phenergan), and the two drugs are equally effective, but ondansetron is much more expensive. No data have been published on first trimester teratogenic risk with ondansetron.

II. **Hyperemesis gravidarum**
   A. Hyperemesis gravidarum occurs in the extreme 0.5% to 1% of patients who have intractable vomiting. Patients with hyperemesis have abnormal electrolytes, dehydration with high urine-specific gravity, ketosis and acetonuria, and untreated have weight loss >5% of body weight. Intravenous hydration is the first line of therapy for patients with severe nausea and vomiting. Administration of vitamin B1 supplements may be necessary to prevent Wernicke's encephalopathy.

B. Antiemetics are given parenterally to patients with hyperemesis. Corticosteroids may have a benefit in hyper-emesis if other antiemetic therapy has failed. One proposed regimen is methylprednisolone 15 to 20 mg given intravenously every 8 hours. A methylprednisolone oral taper regimen is more effective than oral promethazine.

References: See page 166.

Spontaneous Abortion

Abortion is defined as termination of pregnancy resulting in expulsion of an immature, nonviable fetus. A fetus of <20 weeks gestation or a fetus weighing <500 gm is considered an abortus. Spontaneous abortion occurs in 15% of all pregnancies.

I. **Threatened abortion** is defined as vaginal bleeding occurring in the first 20 weeks of pregnancy, without the passage of tissue or rupture of membranes.
  A. Symptoms of pregnancy (nausea, vomiting, fatigue, breast tenderness, urinary frequency) are usually present.
  B. Speculum exam reveals blood coming from the cervical os without amniotic fluid or tissue in the endocervical canal.
  C. The internal cervical os is closed, and the uterus is soft and enlarged appropriate for gestational age.
  D. Differential diagnosis
    1. **Benign and malignant lesions.** The cervix often bleeds from an ectropion of friable tissue. Hemostasis can be accomplished by applying pressure for several minutes with a large swab or by cautery with a silver nitrate stick. Atypical cervical lesions are evaluated with colposcopy and biopsy.
    2. **Disorders of pregnancy**
      a. **Hydatidiform mole** may present with early pregnancy bleeding, passage of grape-like vesicles, and a uterus that is enlarged in excess of that expected from dates. An absence of heart tones by Doppler after 12 weeks is characteristic. Hyperemesis, preeclampsia, or hyperthyroidism may be present. Ultrasonography confirms the diagnosis.
      b. **Ectopic pregnancy** should be excluded when first trimester bleeding is associated with pelvic pain. Orthostatic light-headedness, syncope or shoulder pain (from diaphragmatic irritation) may occur.
        (1) Abdominal tenderness is noted, and pelvic examination reveals cervical motion tenderness.
        (2) Serum beta-HCG is positive.
  E. Laboratory tests
    1. **Complete blood count.** The CBC will not reflect acute blood loss.
    2. **Quantitative serum beta-HCG level** may be positive in nonviable gestations since beta-HCG may persist in the serum for several weeks after fetal death.
    3. **Ultrasonography** should detect fetal heart motion by 7 weeks gestation or older. Failure to detect fetal heart motion after 9 weeks gestation should prompt consideration of curettage.
  F. Treatment of threatened abortion
    1. Bed rest with sedation and abstinence from intercourse.
    2. The patient should report increased bleeding (>normal menses), cramping, passage of tissue, or fever. Passed tissue should be saved for examination.
II. **Inevitable abortion** is defined as a threatened abortion with a dilated cervical os. Menstrual-like cramps usually occur.

    A. Differential diagnosis
        1. Incomplete abortion is diagnosed when tissue has passed. Tissue may be visible in the vagina or endocervical canal.
        2. Threatened abortion is diagnosed when the internal os is closed and will not admit a fingertip.
        3. Incompetent cervix is characterized by dilatation of the cervix without cramps.
    B. Treatment of inevitable abortion
        1. Surgical evacuation of the uterus is necessary.
        2. D immunoglobulin (RhoGAM) is administered to Rh-negative, unsensitized patients to prevent isoimmunization. Before 13 weeks gestation, the dosage is 50 mcg IM; at 13 weeks gestation, the dosage is 300 mcg IM.

III.   **Incomplete abortion** is characterized by cramping, bleeding, passage of tissue, and a dilated internal os with tissue present in the vagina or endocervical canal. Profuse bleeding, orthostatic dizziness, syncope, and postural pulse and blood pressure changes may occur.
    A. Laboratory evaluation
        1. Complete blood count. CBC will not reflect acute blood loss.
        2. Rh typing
        3. Blood typing and cress-matching.
        4. Karyotyping of products of conception is completed if loss is recurrent.
    B. Treatment
        1. Stabilization. If the patient has signs and symptoms of heavy bleeding, at least 2 large-bore IV catheters (<16 gauge) are placed. Lactate Ringer's or normal saline with 40 U oxytocin/L is given IV at 200 mL/hour or greater.
        2. Products of conception are removed from the endocervical canal and uterus with a ring forceps. Immediate removal decreases bleeding. Curettage is performed after vital signs have stabilized.
        3. Suction dilation and curettage
            a. Analgesia consists of meperidine (Demerol), 35-50 mg IV over 3-5 minutes until the patient is drowsy.
            b. The patient is placed in the dorsal lithotomy position in stirrups, prepared, draped, and sedated.
            c. A weighted speculum is placed intravaginally, the vagina and cervix are cleansed, and a paracervical block is placed.
            d. Bimanual examination confirms uterine position and size, and uterine sounding confirms the direction of the endocervical canal.
            e. Mechanical dilatation is completed with dilators if necessary. Curettage is performed with an 8 mm suction curette, with a single-tooth tenaculum on the anterior lip of the cervix.
        4. Post-curettage. After curettage, a blood count is ordered. If the vital signs are stable for several hours, the patient is discharged with instructions to avoid coitus, douching, or the use of tampons for 2 weeks. Ferrous sulfate and ibuprofen are prescribed for pain.
        5. Rh-negative, unsensitized patients are given IM RhoGAM.
        6. Methylergonovine (Methergine), 0.2 mg PO q4h for 6 doses, is given if there is continued moderate bleeding.

IV.   **Complete abortion**
    A. A complete abortion is diagnosed when complete passage of products of conception has occurred. The uterus is well contracted, and the cervical os may be closed.
    B. Differential diagnosis
        1. Incomplete abortion
        2. Ectopic pregnancy. Products of conception should be examined grossly and submitted for pathologic examination. If no fetal tissue or villi are observed grossly, ectopic pregnancy must be excluded by ultrasound.

C. **Management of complete abortion**
  1. Between 8 and 14 weeks, curettage is necessary because of the high probability that the abortion was incomplete.
  2. D immunoglobulin (RhoGAM) is administered to Rh-negative, unsensitized patients.
  3. Beta-HCG levels are obtained weekly until zero. Incomplete abortion is suspected if beta-HCG levels plateau or fail to reach zero within 4 weeks.

V. **Missed abortion** is diagnosed when products of conception are retained after the fetus has expired. If products are retained, a severe coagulopathy with bleeding often occurs.
  A. Missed abortion should be suspected when the pregnant uterus fails to grow as expected or when fetal heart tones disappear.
  B. Amenorrhea may persist, or intermittent vaginal bleeding, spotting, or brown discharge may be noted.
  C. **Ultrasonography** confirms the diagnosis.
  D. **Management of missed abortion**
    1. CBC with platelet count, fibrinogen level, partial thromboplastin time, and ABO blood typing and antibody screen are obtained.
    2. **Evacuation** of the uterus is completed after fetal death has been confirmed. Dilation and evacuation by suction curettage is appropriate when the uterus is less than 12-14 weeks gestational size.
    3. **D immunoglobulin (RhoGAM)** is administered to Rh-negative, unsensitized patients.

References: See page 166.

Urinary Tract Infections in Pregnancy

Urinary tract infection (UTI) is a common problem in pregnancy. Although asymptomatic bacteriuria occurs with equal frequency in pregnant and nonpregnant women, it progresses to symptomatic infection more frequently during pregnancy. The prevalence of asymptomatic bacteriuria is 5 to 9 percent. If asymptomatic bacteriuria is not treated, pyelonephritis will develop in 20 to 40 percent of pregnant patients.

I. **Risk factors for UTI in pregnancy:**
  A. Previous history of UTI, especially before 20 weeks of gestation
  B. Multiparity
  C. Presence of hemoglobin S
  D. Lower socioeconomic status
  E. Sexual activity
  F. Anatomical abnormalities
  G. Diabetes mellitus
  H. Advanced maternal age

II. **Microbiology**. Escherichia coli is responsible for 60 to 90 percent of cases of asymptomatic bacteriuria, cystitis, and pyelonephritis.

III. **Asymptomatic bacteriuria**
  A. Asymptomatic bacteriuria refers to the isolation of $\geq$100,000 CFU of a single organism/mL from a midstream-voided specimen in a woman without UTI symptoms. It occurs in 5 to 9 percent of pregnancies, usually developing in the first month of gestation, particularly in multiparous women.
  B. **Diagnosis**. The definition of a positive urine culture is $\geq 10^5$ CFU/mL.
  C. **Treatment**
    1. **Sulfisoxazole (Gantrisin)** 500 mg PO TID for three days.
    2. **Amoxicillin** 500 mg PO TID for three days.
    3. **Amoxicillin-clavulanate (Augmentin)**, 500 mg PO BID for three days.
    4. **Nitrofurantoin (Macrodantin)** 50 mg PO QID for seven days])
    5. **Cefixime (Suprax)** 250 mg PO QD for three days.

6. **Fosfomycin (Monurol)** 3 g PO as a single dose.
7. These drugs should be used only if the isolate has been established to be susceptible to the agent. Sulfonamides can displace bilirubin from plasma binding sites in the newborn and may cause kernicterus. Sulfonamide therapy is not recommended in the third trimester.
8. **Relapses** typically occur in the first two weeks after treatment and are most common when the bacteriuria originates in the kidney (50 percent). Relapses should be treated with two weeks of oral antibiotics.
9. **Suppressive therapy** is recommended for women with persistent bacteriuria (ie, ≥2 positive urine cultures). Nitrofurantoin (Macrodantin [50 to 100 mg orally at bedtime]) for the duration of the pregnancy or cephalexin (Keflex [250 to 500 mg orally at bedtime]) may be used. A culture for test of cure can be obtained a week after completion of therapy and then repeated monthly until completion of the pregnancy.

IV. **Cystitis**
A. Cystitis occurs in 0.3 to 1.3 percent of pregnant women. Bacteria are confined to the lower urinary tract in these patients.
B. **Clinical features and diagnosis.** Acute cystitis should be considered in any gravida with symptoms of frequency, urgency, dysuria, hematuria, or suprapubic pain in the absence of fever and flank pain. Urine culture is the "gold standard" for diagnosis. However, a CFU count $\geq 10^2$/mL should be considered positive on a midstream urine specimen in women with acute symptoms and pyuria.
C. **Treatment of cystitis**
1. Urine culture should be obtained in patients with signs and symptoms suggestive of cystitis, and empiric antibiotic therapy should be initiated. The treatment should be adjusted depending upon the final culture results and the patient's response to therapy. The same microorganisms associated with asymptomatic bacteriuria are responsible for cystitis.
2. **Amoxicillin** 250 mg TID.
3. **Nitrofurantoin (Macrodantin)** 100 mg BID.
4. **Cephalexin (Keflex)** 500 mg BID to QID.
5. **Amoxicillin-clavulanate (Augmentin)** 500 mg BID or 250 mg TID
6. **Trimethoprim-sulfamethoxazole (Bactrim)** 1 DS BID but not in the third trimester of pregnancy.
7. **Cefpodoxime (Cefzil)** 100 mg BID.
8. **Cefixime (Suprax)** 400 mg QD.
9. All of these drugs can be used for three to seven days. **Monthly urine cultures** should be performed beginning one to two weeks after completion of treatment.

V. **Pyelonephritis**
A. Pyelonephritis complicates 1 to 2 percent of all pregnancies. Seventy-three percent of cases were identified in the antepartum period and 46 percent are diagnosed in the second trimester.
B. **Clinical features and diagnosis.** A combination of fever, chills, and costovertebral angle tenderness is the usual presentation. Other symptoms include dysuria, nausea, vomiting, and respiratory distress.
C. Pyuria is present in virtually all women with this disorder. Urinalysis reveals one or two bacteria per high power field (HPF) in an unspun catheterized specimen or 20 bacteria per HPF in a spun specimen; white cell casts confirm the diagnosis. Urine culture and susceptibility testing are completed.
D. **Complications.** Approximately 20 percent of women with pyelonephritis develop complications such as septic shock, anemia, acute respiratory distress syndrome (ARDS), renal insufficiency, perinephric abscess, and premature labor and birth.
E. **Inpatient treatment**
1. Pyelonephritis in pregnant women is usually treated with hospitalization and intravenous antibiotics until the woman is afebrile for 24 to 48 hours.

2. Parenteral beta lactams or gentamicin are the preferred antibiotics.
   a. Cefazolin (Ancef) 1-2 gm IVPB q8h **OR**
   b. Ampicillin 1 gm IVPB q4-6h **AND**
   c. Gentamicin 2 mg/kg IVPB then 1.5 mg/kg IV q8h **OR**
   d. Ampicillin-sulbactam (Unasyn) 1.5-3 gm IVPB q6h.
3. Symptoms that persist for more than 48 hours, despite adequate intravenous antibiotic therapy, require a renal ultrasound to assess for perinephric abscess or renal calculi.
4. Intravenous treatment should continue until the patient is afebrile for 48 hours. Inpatient therapy is followed by an outpatient course of antibiotics to complete 10 to 14 days of treatment.
5. **Antimicrobial prophylaxis** with nitrofurantoin (Macrodantin [50 to 100 mg PO qhs]) or cephalexin (Keflex [250 to 500 mg PO qhs]), and periodic urinalysis and urine culture are recommended for the remainder of the pregnancy.
F. **Outpatient treatment** may be considered in the setting of uncomplicated disease (eg, absence of underlying medical conditions, anatomic abnormalities, pregnancy complications, or signs of sepsis).

References: See page 166.

Trauma During Pregnancy

Trauma is the leading cause of nonobstetric death in women of reproductive age. Six percent of all pregnancies are complicated by some type of trauma.

I. Mechanism of injury
   A. Blunt abdominal trauma
      1. Blunt abdominal trauma secondary to motor vehicle accidents is the leading cause of nonobstetric-related fetal death during pregnancy, followed by falls and assaults. Uterine rupture or laceration, retroperitoneal hemorrhage, renal injury and upper abdominal injuries may also occur after blunt trauma.
      2. **Abruptio placentae** occurs in 40-50% of patients with major traumatic injuries and in up to 5% of patients with minor injuries.
      3. **Clinical findings in blunt abdominal trauma.** Vaginal bleeding, uterine tenderness, uterine contractions, fetal tachycardia, late decelerations, fetal acidosis, and fetal death.
      4. **Detection of abruptio placentae.** Beyond 20 weeks of gestation, external electronic monitoring can detect uterine contractile activity. The presence of vaginal bleeding and tetanic or hypertonic contractions is presumptive evidence of abruptio placentae.
      5. **Uterine rupture**
         a. Uterine rupture is an infrequent but life-threatening complication. It usually occurs after a direct abdominal impact.
         b. Findings of uterine rupture range from subtle (uterine tenderness, nonreassuring fetal heart rate pattern) to severe, with rapid onset of maternal hypovolemic shock and death.
      6. **Direct fetal injury** is an infrequent complication of blunt trauma.
         a. The fetus is more frequently injured as a result of hypoxia from blood loss or abruption.
         b. In the first trimester the uterus is well protected by the maternal pelvis; therefore, minor trauma usually does not usually cause miscarriage in the first trimester.
   B. Penetrating trauma
      1. Penetrating abdominal trauma from gunshot and stab wounds during pregnancy has a poor prognosis.
      2. Perinatal mortality is 41-71%. Maternal mortality is less than 5%.
II. Major trauma in pregnancy
   A. **Initial evaluation of major abdominal trauma** in pregnant patients does not differ from evaluation of abdominal trauma in a nonpregnant patient.

B. **Maintain airway, breathing, and circulatory volume.** Two large-bore (14-16-gauge) intravenous lines are placed.

C. **Oxygen** should be administered by mask or endotracheal intubation. Maternal oxygen saturation should be kept at >90% (an oxygen partial pressure [pO_2] of 60 mm Hg).

D. **Volume resuscitation**
   1. Crystalloid in the form of lactated Ringer's or normal saline should be given as a 3:1 replacement for the estimated blood loss over the first 30-60 minutes of acute resuscitation.
   2. O-negative packed red cells are preferred if emergent blood is needed before the patient's own blood type is known.
   3. A urinary catheter should be placed to measure urine output and observe for hematuria.

E. **Deflection of the uterus** off the inferior vena cava and abdominal aorta can be achieved by placing the patient in the lateral decubitus position. If the patient must remain supine, manual deflection of the uterus to the left and placement of a wedge under the patient's hip or backboard will tilt the patient.

F. **Secondary survey.** Following stabilization, a more detailed secondary survey of the patient, including fetal evaluation, is performed.

III. **Minor trauma in pregnancy**
   A. **Clinical evaluation**
      1. Pregnant patients who sustain seemingly minimal trauma require an evaluation to exclude significant injuries. Common "minor" trauma include falls, especially in the third trimester, blows to the abdomen, and "fender benders" motor vehicle accidents.
      2. The patient should be questioned about seat belt use, loss of consciousness, pain, vaginal bleeding, rupture of membranes, and fetal movement.
      3. **Physical examination**
         a. Physical examination should focus on upper abdominal tenderness (liver or spleen damage), flank pain (renal trauma), uterine pain (placental abruption, uterine rupture), and pain over the symphysis pubis (pelvic fracture, bladder laceration, fetal skull fracture).
         b. A search for orthopedic injuries should be completed.
   B. **Management of minor trauma**
      1. The minor trauma patient with a fetus that is less than 20 weeks gestation (not yet viable), with no significant injury can be safely discharged after documentation of fetal heart rate. Patients with potentially viable fetuses (over 20 weeks of gestation) require fetal monitoring, laboratory tests and ultrasonographic evaluation.
      2. A complete blood count, urinalysis (hematuria), blood type and screen (to check Rh status), and coagulation panel, including measurement of the INR, PTT, fibrinogen and fibrin split products, should be obtained. The coagulation panel is useful if any suspicion of abruption exists.
      3. **The Kleihauer-Betke (KB) test**
         a. This test detects fetal red blood cells in the maternal circulation. A KB stain should be obtained routinely for any pregnant trauma patient whose fetus is over 12 weeks.
         b. Regardless of the patient's blood type and Rh status, the KB test can help determine if fetomaternal hemorrhage has occurred.
         c. The KB test can also be used to determine the amount of Rho(D) immunoglobulin (RhoGAM) required in patients who are Rh-negative.
         d. A positive KB stain indicates uterine trauma, and any patient with a positive KB stain should receive at least 24 hours of continuous uterine and fetal monitoring and a coagulation panel.
      4. **Ultrasonography** is less sensitive for diagnosing abruption than is the finding of uterine contractions on external tocodynamometry. Absence of sonographic evidence of abruption does not completely exclude an abruption.

5. Patients with abdominal pain, significant bruising, vaginal bleeding, rupture of membranes, or uterine contractions should be admitted to the hospital for overnight observation and continuous fetal monitor.

6. Uterine contractions and vaginal bleeding are suggestive of abruption. Even if vaginal bleeding is absent, the presence of contractions is still a concern, since the uterus can contain up to 2 L of blood from a concealed abruption.

7. Trauma patients with no uterine contraction activity, usually do not have abruption, while patients with greater than one contraction per 10 minutes (6 per hour) have a 20% incidence of abruption.

References: See page 166.

Gestational Diabetes Mellitus

Poorly controlled gestational diabetes is associated with an increase in the incidence of preeclampsia, polyhydramnios, fetal macrosomia, birth trauma, operative delivery, and neonatal hypoglycemia. There is an increased incidence of hyperbilirubinemia, hypocalcemia, and erythremia. The perinatal mortality is increased, as is the likelihood of development of obesity and diabetes in offspring during childhood. Later development of diabetes mellitus in the mother is also more frequent. The prevalence of gestational diabetes is higher in black, Hispanic, Native American, and Asian women than white women. The prevalence of gestational diabetes is 1.4 to 14 percent.

Risk Factors for Gestational Diabetes
• A family history of diabetes, especially in first degree relatives
• Prepregnancy weight of 110 percent of ideal body weight (pregravid weight more than 90 kg) or more or weight gain in early adulthood.
• Age greater than 25 years
• A previous large baby (greater than 9 pounds [4.1 kg])
• History of abnormal glucose tolerance
• Hispanic, African, Native American, South or East Asian, and Pacific Island ancestry
• A previous unexplained perinatal loss or birth of a malformed child
• The mother was large at birth (greater than 9 pounds [4.1 kg])
• Polycystic ovary syndrome

I. **Screening and diagnostic criteria**
   A. Screening for gestational diabetes should be performed at 24 to 28 weeks of gestation. However, it can be done as early as the first prenatal visit if there is a high degree of suspicion that the pregnant woman has undiagnosed type 2 diabetes (eg, obesity, previous gestational diabetes or fetal macrosomia, age >25 years, family history of diabetes).
   B. **50-g oral glucose challenge** is given and venous serum or plasma glucose is measured one hour later; a value ≥140 mg/dL (7.8 mmol/L) is considered abnormal. Women with an abnormal value are then given a 100-g, three-hour oral glucose tolerance test (GTT).

Criteria for Gestational Diabetes with Three Hour Oral Glucose Tolerance Test	
Fasting	>95 mg/dL
1 hour	>180 mg/dL
2 hour	>155 mg/dL
3 hour	>140 mg/dL
Any two or more abnormal results are diagnostic of gestational diabetes.	

II. Treatment of gestational diabetes mellitus

A. Diet

1. Dietary therapy should be started in women who do not meet criteria for gestational diabetes (abnormal glucose tolerance test) if they have fasting blood glucose concentrations >90 mg/dL or an abnormal glucose challenge test.

2. **Caloric intake**
   a. **Pregnant women who are 80 to 120 percent of ideal body weight:** 30 kcal per present weight in kg per day.
   b. **Overweight pregnant women (120 to 150 percent of ideal body weight):** 24 kcal per present weight in kg per day.
   c. **Morbidly obese pregnant women (>150 percent of ideal body weight):** 12 to 15 kcal per present weight in kg per day.
   d. **Pregnant women who are less than 80 percent of ideal body weight:** 40 kcal per present weight in kg per day.

3. **Calorie distribution**: 40 percent carbohydrate, 20 percent protein, and 40 percent fat.
   a. With this calorie distribution, 75 to 80 percent of women with gestational diabetes can achieve normoglycemia.
   b. Three meals and three snacks per day are recommended. Breakfast must be very small (10 percent of total calories) to prevent the blood glucose concentration one hour after breakfast from rising above 120 mg/dL. The remaining calories should be distributed as 30 percent at both lunch and dinner, with the leftover calories distributed as snacks.

Treatment Goals for Gestational Diabetes Mellitus	
Time	**Blood Sugar**
Fasting	<90 mg/dL
1 hr postprandial	<120 mg/dL

B. Initiation of insulin therapy

1. Approximately 15 percent of women with gestational diabetes require insulin because of elevated blood glucose despite dietary therapy.

2. Insulin should be initiated when the fasting blood glucose concentration is greater than 90 mg/dL and the one-hour postprandial blood glucose concentration is greater than 120 mg/dL on two or more occasions within a two-week interval despite dietary therapy.

3. **Insulin regimen**
   a. If insulin is required because the fasting blood glucose concentration is high, an intermediate-acting insulin, such as NPH insulin, is given before bedtime. The initial dose should be 0.15 U/kg body

weight.
   b. If postprandial blood glucose concentrations are high, then regular insulin or insulin lispro should be given before meals at 1.5 U per 10 grams carbohydrate in the breakfast meal and 1.0 U per 10 grams carbohydrate in the lunch and dinner meals.
   c. If both preprandial and postprandial blood glucose concentrations are high, then a four-injection per day regimen should be initiated. The total dose is 0.7 U/kg for weeks six to 18, 0.8 U/kg for weeks 19 to 26, 0.9 U/kg for weeks 27 to 36, and 1.0 U/kg for weeks 37 to term.
   d. The insulin should be divided as 45 percent as NPH insulin, 30 percent before breakfast and 15 percent before bedtime, and about 55 percent as preprandial regular insulin, 22 percent before breakfast, 16.5 percent before lunch, and 16.5 percent before dinner. Insulin resistance increases as gestation proceeds, requiring an increase in insulin dose.

C. Fetal surveillance
   1. Fetal surveillance should be initiated in the third trimester in women in whom gestational diabetes is not well-controlled, who require insulin, or have other complications of pregnancy (eg, hypertension). Counting fetal movements is a simple way to assess fetal well-being. Fewer than ten fetal movements in a 12-hour period is associated with a poor outcome.
   2. Early delivery. Women with good glycemic control and no other complications of pregnancy ideally will deliver at 39 to 40 weeks of gestation. Indications for delivery before the 39th week include poor glycemic control and fetal abnormalities. If early delivery is indicated, lung maturity should be assessed by amniocentesis if delivery could be safely postponed in the absence of fetal pulmonary maturity.
   3. Normal delivery. The great majority of women with gestational diabetes proceed to term and have a spontaneous vaginal delivery. The maternal blood glucose concentration should be maintained between 70 and 90 mg/dL. Insulin can usually be withheld during delivery, and an infusion of normal saline is usually sufficient to maintain normoglycemia.

Low-dosage Constant Insulin Infusion for the Intrapartum Period		
Blood Glucose (mg/100 mL)	**Insulin Dosage (U/h)**	**Fluids (125 mL/h)**
<100	0	5%dextrose/Lactated Ringer's solution
100-140	1.0	5% dextrose/Lactated Ringer's solution
141-180	1.5	Normal saline
181-220	2.0	Normal saline
>220	2.5	Normal saline

Dilution is 25 U of regular insulin in 250 mL of normal saline, with 25 mL flushed through line, administered intravenously.

D. Postpartum concerns and follow-up
   1. Nearly all women with gestational diabetes are normoglycemic after delivery. However, they are at risk for gestational diabetes, impaired glucose tolerance, and overt diabetes.

2. Immediately after delivery, blood glucose should be measured to ensure that the mother no longer has hyperglycemia. Fasting blood glucose concentrations should be below 115 mg/dL and one-hour postprandial concentrations should be below 140 mg/dL.

References: See page 166.

Diabetes Mellitus

Approximately 4 percent of pregnant women have diabetes: 88 percent have gestational diabetes mellitus, while the remaining 12 percent have pregestational diabetes. Of those with pregestational diabetes, 35 percent have type 1 and 65 percent type 2 diabetes.

I. **Glycemic control and fetal and maternal complications**
   A. Pregnancy in diabetes is associated with an increase in risk of congenital anomalies and spontaneous abortions in women who are in poor glycemic control during the period of fetal organogenesis, which is nearly complete at seven weeks postconception.
   B. **Macrosomia.** Another consequence of poor glycemic control in pregnant women with diabetes is fetal macrosomia, which leads to dystocia, an increased need for cesarean delivery, and an increase in fetal morbidity.
   C. **Glucose monitoring**. Frequent measurements of blood glucose are mandatory in women with type 1 diabetes during pregnancy. If the first morning blood glucose value is high, testing should also be performed at bedtime and in middle of the night.

Testing during Pregnancy in Type I Diabetes	
Test	**Frequency**
Hemoglobin A1c	Every 4-6 weeks
Blood glucose	4-8 times daily at home; during weekly/biweekly visits' in physician's office
Urine ketones	During period of illness; when any blood glucose value is ≥200 mg/dL
Urinalysis	Weekly/biweekly office visits
Serum creatinine	Each trimester
Thyroid function tests	Baseline measurements of serum free T4 and TSH
Eye examination	At baseline and as necessary per retinal specialist

   D. **Urinary ketones** should be measured periodically, especially when the woman is ill or when any blood glucose value is over 200 mg/dL. At these times ketoacidosis may occur, a complication that is associated with a high mortality rate in the fetus.
   E. **Target blood glucose values**
      1. **Hemoglobin A1c (HbA1c)** should be measured every four to six weeks and more frequently if the woman's glycemic control is poor.
      2. **Blood glucose goals in a pregnant diabetic:**
         a. **Fasting capillary blood glucose** concentration of 55 to 65 mg/dL, about 85 percent for the venous plasma concentration.
         b. **One-hour postprandial blood glucose** concentration less than 120 mg/dL.

F. **Recommendations for caloric intake:**
   1. **Woman at ideal body weight:** 30 kcal/kg per day.
   2. **20 to 50 percent above ideal body weight:** 24 kcal/kg per day.
   3. **More than 50 percent above ideal body weight:** 12 to 18 kcal/kg per day.
   4. **More than 10 percent below ideal body weight:** 36 to 40 kcal/day.
G. **Recommended distribution of calories:** 40 to 50 percent carbohydrate, 20 percent protein, and 30 to 40 percent fat. Patients should eat three meals and three snacks per day. The calorie distribution should be 10 percent of calories at breakfast, 30 percent at both lunch and dinner, and 30 percent as snacks. A daily supplement of ferrous sulfate (30 mg) and folate (400 µg) is also recommended.
H. **Insulin regimen**
   1. Most women with type 1 diabetes require at least three injections of insulin per day. After an early rise in insulin requirements between weeks 3 and 7, there often is a significant decline between weeks 7 and 15, followed by a rise during the remainder of pregnancy.
   2. The average insulin requirement in pregnant women with type 1 diabetes is 0.7 units/kg in the first trimester, often increasing to 0.8 U/kg for weeks 18 to 26, 0.9 U/kg for weeks 27 to 36, and 1.0 U/kg for weeks 37 to term.

Insulin Adjustment Based on Blood Glucose (BG)

Time	Insulin dose being adjusted	Adjustment
7:30 AM	Bedtime NPH	If BG is >90 mg/dL, check at bedtime and 3:00 AM. If bedtime value is high, increase dinner regular insulin. If bedtime value normal but 3:00 AM value is above 100 mg/dL, then raise bedtime NPH by 2 units. If 3:00 AM value is below 60 mg/dL, then decrease bedtime NPH by 2 units. If 7:30 AM value is below 60 mg/dL, reduce bedtime NPH by 2 units.
10:00 AM	Morning regular	If 1 hour postprandial is above 140 mg/dL, increase next morning regular insulin by 2 units. If the value is <110 mg/dL, decrease next morning AM regular by 2 units.
1:00 PM	Lunch regular	If 1 hour postprandial value is above 140 mg/dL, increase lunch regular insulin for the next day by 2 units. If the value Is below 110 mg/dL, decrease next day's lunch regular insulin by 2 units.
4:30 PM	Morning NPH	If BG is above 90 mg/dL, then increase morning NPH by 2 units. If 90 is below 60 mg/dL, then decrease morning NPH by 2 units.
6:00 PM	Dinner regular	If 1 hour postprandial value is above 140 mg/dL, increase dinner regular insulin by 2 units. If 1 hour value is below 110 mg/dL, decrease dinner regular insulin by 2 units.

   3. Women with type 2 diabetes also should be treated with insulin. During the first trimester, insulin requirements are similar in women with type 1 and type 2 diabetes. However, as the pregnancy proceeds into the third trimester, insulin requirements increase proportionately more in women with type 2 than type 1 diabetes.

4. A combination of regular insulin and intermediate-acting insulin (such as NPH insulin) should be administered. The insulin is initially distributed as follows:
   a. 45 percent of the total daily dose is given as NPH insulin and 22 percent as regular insulin before breakfast.
   b. 17 percent of the total daily dose is given as both NPH and regular insulin before dinner.
   c. The premeal dose of regular insulin is given on a sliding scale according to the blood glucose value.
5. **Macrosomia** is defined as fetal weight greater than 4.0 to 4.5 kg or birth weight above the 90th percentile for gestational age. Macrosomic fetuses are at increased risk for a prolonged second stage of labor, shoulder dystocia, operative delivery, and perinatal death.
6. **Congenital anomalies**. Ultrasonography is essential for the evaluation of congenital anomalies. Congenital anomalies that occur with higher frequency include anencephaly, microcephaly, caudal regression syndrome, and genitourinary and gastrointestinal anomalies. Congenital heart disease may include hypertrophic cardiomyopathy, atrial and ventricular septal defects, transposition of the great vessels and coarctation of the aorta.
7. **Polyhydramnios** can occur because of increased amniotic fluid osmolality and polyuria secondary to fetal hyperglycemia.
8. **Antepartum surveillance.** In women with diet-controlled gestational diabetes, fetal surveillance is usually not initiated until 40 weeks gestation, since these women are at very low risk for complications. More rigorous monitoring is recommended for women who have additional indications for closer fetal surveillance, such as hypertension. Surveillance begins earlier in women with either gestational or pregestational diabetes treated with insulin. Testing is begun at the 35th week of gestation if there is excellent glycemic control. Testing should start at 26 to 28 weeks in women with poor control, nephropathy, or hypertension.

I. **Labor and delivery**
   1. Insulin is required before active labor and can be given subcutaneously or by intravenous infusion with a goal of maintaining blood glucose concentrations between 70 and 90 mg/dL. The insulin infusion consists of administration of 15 units of regular insulin in 150 mL of normal saline IV at a rate of one to three units per hour.
   2. Normal saline may be sufficient to maintain euglycemia when labor is anticipated.
   3. When active labor begins, insulin resistance rapidly decreases and insulin requirements fall rapidly. Thus, continuing insulin therapy is likely to lead to hypoglycemia. To prevent this, glucose should be infused at a rate of 2.5 mg/kg per min. Capillary blood glucose should be measured hourly. The glucose infusion should be doubled for the next hour if the blood glucose value is less than 60 mg/dL. However if the value is 120 mg/dL or more, regular insulin is given subcutaneously or intravenously until the blood glucose value falls to 70 to 90 mg/dL. The insulin dose is titrated to maintain normoglycemia while glucose is infused at a rate of 2.5 mg/kg per min.
   4. If a cesarean section is planned, the bedtime NPH insulin dose may be given on the morning of surgery and every eight hours thereafter if surgery is delayed.
   5. Insulin requirements drop sharply after delivery, and the new mother may not require insulin for 24 to 72 hours. Insulin requirements should be recalculated at this time at 0.6 units/kg per day based upon postpartum weight. Postpartum calorie requirements are approximately 25 kcal/kg per day, and 27 kcal/kg per day in lactating women.
   6. Women in whom labor is induced should receive no morning insulin. Blood glucose monitoring and glucose and insulin infusion are managed as for active labor.

References: See page 166.

Group B Streptococcal Infection in Pregnancy

Group B streptococcus (GBS; Streptococcus agalactiae), a Gram positive coccus, is an important cause of infection in neonates, causing sepsis, pneumonia, and meningitis. GBS infection is acquired in utero or during passage through the vagina. Vaginal colonization with GBS during pregnancy may lead to premature birth, and GBS is a frequent cause of maternal urinary tract infection, chorioamnionitis, postpartum endometritis, and bacteremia.

I. **Clinical evaluation**
   A. The primary risk factor for GBS infection is maternal GBS genitourinary or gastrointestinal colonization.
   B. The rate of transmission from colonized mothers to infants is approximately 50 percent. However, only 1 to 2 percent of all colonized infants develop early-onset GBS disease.
   C. **Maternal obstetrical factors associated with neonatal GBS disease:**
      1. Delivery at less than 37 weeks of gestation
      2. Premature rupture of membranes
      3. Rupture of membranes for 18 or more hours before delivery
      4. Chorioamnionitis
      5. Temperature greater than 38°C during labor
      6. Sustained intrapartum fetal tachycardia
      7. Prior delivery of an infant with GBS disease
   D. **Manifestations of early-onset GBS disease.** Early-onset disease results in bacteremia, generalized sepsis, pneumonia, or meningitis. The clinical signs usually are apparent in the first hours of life.
II. **2002 CDC guidelines for intrapartum antibiotic prophylaxis:**
   A. All pregnant women should be screened for GBS colonization with swabs of both the lower vagina and rectum at 35 to 37 weeks of gestation. Patients are excluded from screening if they had GBS bacteriuria earlier in the pregnancy or if they gave birth to a previous infant with invasive GBS disease. These latter patients should receive intrapartum antibiotic prophylaxis regardless of the colonization status.
   B. **Intrapartum antibiotic prophylaxis is recommended for the following:**
      1. Pregnant women with a positive screening culture unless a planned Cesarean section is performed in the absence of labor or rupture of membranes
      2. Pregnant women who gave birth to a previous infant with invasive GBS disease
      3. Pregnant women with documented GBS bacteriuria during the current pregnancy
      4. Pregnant women whose culture status is unknown (culture not performed or result not available) and who also have delivery at <37 weeks of gestation, amniotic membrane rupture for ≥18 hours, or intrapartum temperature ≥100.4°F (≥38°C)
   C. **Intrapartum antibiotic prophylaxis is not recommended for the following patients:**
      1. Positive GBS screening culture in a previous pregnancy (unless the infant had invasive GBS disease or the screening culture is also positive in the current pregnancy)
      2. Patient who undergoes a planned Cesarean section without labor or rupture of membranes
      3. Pregnant women with negative GBS screening cultures at 35 to 37 weeks of gestation even if they have one or more of the above intrapartum risk factors
   D. **Recommended IAP regimen**
      1. **Penicillin G** (5 million units IV initial dose, then 2.5 million units IV Q4h) is recommended for most patients.

    2. **In women with non-immediate-type penicillin-allergy,** cefazolin (Ancef, 2 g initial dose, then 1 g Q8h) is recommended.

    3. **Patients at high risk for anaphylaxis to penicillins** are treated with clindamycin (900 mg IV Q8h) or erythromycin (500 mg IV Q6h) as long as their GBS isolate is documented to be susceptible to both clindamycin and erythromycin.

    4. **For patients at high risk for anaphylaxis and a GBS resistant isolate** (or with unknown susceptibility) to clindamycin or erythromycin, vancomycin (1 g Q12h) should be given.

    5. Antibiotic therapy is continued from hospital admission through delivery.

  E. Approach to threatened preterm delivery at <37 weeks of gestation: A patient with negative GBS cultures (after 35 weeks of gestation) should not be treated during threatened labor. If GBS cultures have not been performed, these specimens should be obtained and penicillin G administered as above; if cultures are negative at 48 hours, penicillin can be discontinued. If such a patient has not delivered within four weeks, cultures should be repeated.

  F. If screening cultures taken at the time of threatened delivery or previously performed (after 35 weeks of gestation) are positive, penicillin should be continued for at least 48 hours unless delivery supervenes. Patients who have been treated for ≥48 hours and have not delivered should receive IAP as above when delivery occurs.

References: See page 166.

Premature Rupture of Membranes

Premature rupture of membranes (PROM) is the most common diagnosis associated with preterm delivery. The incidence of this disorder to be 7-12%. In pregnancies of less than 37 weeks of gestation, preterm birth (and its sequelae) and infection are the major concerns after PROM.

I. Pathophysiology

  A. Premature rupture of membranes is defined as rupture of membranes prior to the onset of labor.

  B. Preterm premature rupture of membranes is defined as rupture of membranes prior to term.

  C. Prolonged rupture of membranes consists of rupture of membranes for more than 24 hours.

  D. The latent period is the time interval from rupture of membranes to the onset of regular contractions or labor.

  E. Many cases of preterm PROM are caused by idiopathic weakening of the membranes, many of which are caused by subclinical infection. Other causes of PROM include hydramnios, incompetent cervix, abruptio placentae, and amniocentesis.

  F. At term, about 8% of patients will present with ruptured membranes prior to the onset of labor.

II. Maternal and neonatal complications

  A. Labor usually follows shortly after the occurrence of PROM. Ninety percent of term patients and 50% of preterm patients go into labor within 24 hours after rupture.

  B. Patients who do not go into labor immediately are at increasing risk of infection as the duration of rupture increases. Chorioamnionitis, endometritis, sepsis, and neonatal infections may occur.

  C. Perinatal risks with preterm PROM are primarily complications from immaturity, including respiratory distress syndrome, intraventricular hemorrhage, patent ductus arteriosus, and necrotizing enterocolitis.

  D. Premature gestational age is a more significant cause of neonatal morbidity than is the duration of membrane rupture.

III. **Diagnosis of premature rupture of membranes**
   A. Diagnosis is based on history, physical examination, and laboratory testing. The patient's history alone is correct in 90% of patients. Urinary leakage or excess vaginal discharge is sometimes mistaken for PROM.
   B. **Sterile speculum exam** is the first step in confirming the suspicion of PROM. Digital examination should be avoided because it increases the risk of infection.
      1. The general appearance of the cervix should be assessed visually, and prolapse of the umbilical cord or a fetal extremity should be excluded. Cultures for group B streptococcus, gonorrhea, and chlamydia are obtained.
      2. A pool of fluid in the posterior vaginal fornix supports the diagnosis of PROM.
      3. The presence of amniotic fluid is confirmed by nitrazine testing for an alkaline pH. Amniotic fluid causes nitrazine paper to turn dark blue because the pH is above 6.0-6.5. Nitrazine may be false-positive with contamination from blood, semen, or vaginitis.
      4. If pooling and nitrazine are both non-confirmatory, a swab from the posterior fornix should be smeared on a slide, allowed to dry, and examined under a microscope for "ferning," indicating amniotic fluid.
      5. Ultrasound examination for oligohydramnios is useful to confirm the diagnosis, but oligohydramnios may be caused by other disorders besides PROM.

IV. **Assessment of premature rupture of membranes**
   A. The gestational age must be carefully assessed. Menstrual history, prenatal exams, and previous sonograms are reviewed. An ultrasound examination should be performed.
   B. The patient should be evaluated for the presence of chorioamnionitis [fever (over 38°C), leukocytosis, maternal and fetal tachycardia, uterine tenderness, foul-smelling vaginal discharge].
   C. The patient should be evaluated for labor, and a sterile speculum examination should assess cervical change.
   D. The fetus should be evaluated with heart rate monitoring because PROM increases the risk of umbilical cord prolapse and fetal distress caused by oligohydramnios.

V. **Management of premature rupture of membranes**
   A. **Term patients**
      1. At 36 weeks and beyond, management of PROM consists of delivery. Patients in active labor should be allowed to progress.
      2. Patients with chorioamnionitis, who are not in labor, should be immediately induced with oxytocin (Pitocin).
      3. Patients who are not yet in active labor (in the absence of fetal distress, meconium, or clinical infection) may be discharged for 48 hours, and labor usually follows. If labor has not begun within a reasonable time after rupture of membranes, induction with oxytocin (Pitocin) is appropriate. Use of prostaglandin E2 is safe for cervical ripening.
   B. **Preterm patients**
      1. Preterm patients with PROM prior to 36 weeks are managed expectantly. Delivery is delayed for the patients who are not in labor, not infected, and without evidence of fetal distress.
      2. Patients should be monitored for infection. Cultures for gonococci, Chlamydia, and group B streptococci are obtained. Symptoms, vital signs, uterine tenderness, odor of the lochia, and leukocyte counts are monitored.
      3. Suspected occult chorioamnionitis is diagnosed by amniocentesis for Gram stain and culture, which will reveal gram positive cocci in chains.
      4. Ultrasound examination should be performed to detect oligohydramnios.

5. **Intrapartum antibiotic prophylaxis group B streptococcal is recommended for the following:**
   a. Pregnant women with a positive screening culture unless a planned Cesarean section is performed in the absence of labor or rupture of membranes
   b. Pregnant women who gave birth to a previous infant with invasive GBS disease
   c. Pregnant women with documented GBS bacteriuria during the current pregnancy
   d. Pregnant women whose culture status is unknown (culture not performed or result not available) and who also have delivery at <37 weeks of gestation, amniotic membrane rupture for ≥18 hours, or intrapartum temperature ≥100.4°F (≥38°C)
   e. The recommended IAP regimen is penicillin G (5 million units IV initial dose, then 2.5 million units IV Q4h). In women with non-immediate-type penicillin-allergy, cefazolin (Ancef, 2 g initial dose, then 1 g Q8h) is recommended.
6. Prolonged continuous fetal heart rate monitoring in the initial assessment should be followed by frequent fetal evaluation.
7. Premature labor is the most common outcome of preterm PROM. Tocolytic drugs are often used and corticosteroids are recommended to accelerate fetal pulmonary maturity.
8. Expectant management consists of in-hospital observation. Delivery is indicated for chorioamnionitis, irreversible fetal distress, or premature labor. Once gestation reaches 36 weeks, the patient may be managed as any other term patient with PROM. Another option is to evaluate the fetus at less than 36 weeks for pulmonary maturity and expedite delivery once maturity is documented by testing of amniotic fluid collected by amniocentesis or from the vagina. A positive phosphatidylglycerol test indicates fetal lung maturity.

C. **Previable or preterm premature rupture of membranes**
   1. In patients in whom membranes rupture very early in pregnancy (eg, <25 weeks). There is a relatively low likelihood (<25%) that a surviving infant will be delivered, and infants that do survive will deliver very premature and suffer significant morbidity.
   2. **Fetal deformation syndrome.** The fetus suffering from prolonged early oligohydramnios may develop pulmonary hypoplasia, facial deformation, limb contractures, and deformity.
   3. Termination of pregnancy is advisable if the gestational age is early. If the patient elects to continue the pregnancy, expectant management with pelvic rest at home is reasonable.

D. **Chorioamnionitis**
   1. Chorioamnionitis requires delivery (usually vaginally), regardless of the gestational age.
   2. **Antibiotic therapy**
      a. Ampicillin 2 gm IV q4-6h **AND**
      b. Gentamicin 100 mg (2 mg/kg) IV load, then 100 mg (1.5 mg/kg) IV q8h.

References: See page 166.

Preterm Labor

Preterm labor is the leading cause of perinatal morbidity and mortality in the United States. It usually results in preterm birth, a complication that affects 8 to 10 percent of births.

Risk Factors for Preterm Labor	

Previous preterm delivery
Low socioeconomic status
Non-white race
Maternal age <18 years or >40 years
Preterm premature rupture of the membranes
Multiple gestation
Maternal history of one or more spontaneous second-trimester abortions
Maternal complications
  --Maternal behaviors
  --Smoking
  --Illicit drug use
  --Alcohol use
  --Lack of prenatal care
Uterine causes
  --Myomata (particularly submucosal or subplacental)
  --Uterine septum
  --Bicornuate uterus
  --Cervical incompetence
  --Exposure to diethylstilbestrol (DES)
	Infectious causes
	  --Chorioamnionitis
	  --Bacterial vaginosis
	  --Asymptomatic bacteriuria
	  --Acute pyelonephritis
	  --Cervical/vaginal colonization
	Fetal causes
	  --Intrauterine fetal death
	  --Intrauterine growth retardation
	  --Congenital anomalies
	Abnormal placentation
	Presence of a retained intrauterine device

I. **Risk factors for preterm labor.** Preterm labor is characterized by cervical effacement and/or dilatation, and increased uterine irritability that occurs before 37 weeks of gestation. Women with a history of previous preterm delivery carry the highest risk of recurrence, estimated to be between 17 and 37 percent.

II. **Management of preterm labor**
  A. **Tocolysis**
    1. Tocolytic therapy may offer some short-term benefit in the management of preterm labor. A delay in delivery can be used to administer corticosteroids to enhance pulmonary maturity and reduce the severity of fetal respiratory distress syndrome, and to reduce the risk of intraventricular hemorrhage. No study has convincingly demonstrated an improvement in survival or neonatal outcome with the use of tocolytic therapy alone.
    2. Contraindications to tocolysis include nonreassuring fetal heart rate tracing, eclampsia or severe preeclampsia, fetal demise (singleton), chorioamnionitis, fetal maturity and maternal hemodynamic instability.
    3. Tocolytic therapy is indicated for regular uterine contractions and cervical change (effacement or dilatation). Oral terbutaline (Bricanyl) following successful parenteral tocolysis is not associated with prolonged pregnancy or reduced incidence of recurrent preterm labor.

Preterm Labor, Threatened or Actual

1. Initial assessment to determine whether patient is experiencing preterm labor
   a. Assess for the following:
      i. Uterine activity
      ii. Rupture of membranes
      iii. Vaginal bleeding
      iv. Presentation
      v. Cervical dilation and effacement
      vi. Station
   b. Reassess estimate of gestational age
2. Search for a precipitating factor/cause
3. Consider specific management strategies, which may include the following:
   a. Intravenous tocolytic therapy (decision should be influenced by gestational age, cause of preterm labor and contraindications)
   b. Corticosteroid therapy (eg, betamethasone, in a dosage of 12 mg IM every 24 hours for a total of two doses)
   c. Antibiotic therapy if specific infectious agent is identified or if preterm premature rupture of the membranes

Tocolytic Therapy for the Management of Preterm Labor

Medication	Mechanism of action	Dosage
Magnesium sulfate	Intracellular calcium antagonism	4 to 6 g loading dose; then 2 to 4 g IV every hour
Terbutaline (Bricanyl)	Beta₂-adrenergic receptor agonist sympathomimetic; decreases free intracellular calcium ions	0.25 to 0.5 mg SC every three to four hours
Ritodrine (Yutopar)	Same as terbutaline	0.05 to 0.35 mg per minute IV
Nifedipine (Procardia)	Calcium channel blocker	5 to 10 mg SL every 15 to 20 minutes (up to four times), then 10 to 20 mg orally every four to six hours
Indomethacin (Indocin)	Prostaglandin inhibitor	50- to 100-mg rectal suppository, then 25 to 50 mg orally every six hours

Complications Associated With the Use of Tocolytic Agents

Magnesium sulfate
- Pulmonary edema
- Profound hypotension
- Profound muscular paralysis
- Maternal tetany
- Cardiac arrest
- Respiratory depression

Beta-adrenergic agents
- Hypokalemia
- Hyperglycemia
- Hypotension
- Pulmonary edema
- Arrhythmias
- Cardiac insufficiency
- Myocardial ischemia
- Maternal death

Indomethacin (Indocin)
- Renal failure
- Hepatitis
- Gastrointestinal bleeding

Nifedipine (Procardia)
- Transient hypotension

B. Corticosteroid therapy
1. Dexamethasone and betamethasone are the preferred corticosteroids for antenatal therapy. Corticosteroid therapy for fetal maturation reduces mortality, respiratory distress syndrome and intraventricular hemorrhage in infants between 24 and 34 weeks of gestation.
2. In women with preterm premature rupture of membranes (PPROM), antenatal corticosteroid therapy reduces the risk of respiratory distress syndrome. In women with PPROM at less than 30 to 32 weeks of gestation, in the absence of clinical chorioamnionitis, antenatal corticosteroid use is recommended because of the high risk of intraventricular hemorrhage at this early gestational age.

Recommended Antepartum Corticosteroid Regimens for Fetal Maturation in Preterm Infants

Medication	Dosage
Betamethasone (Celestone)	12 mg IM every 24 hours for two doses
Dexamethasone	6 mg IM every 12 hours for four doses

C. Intrapartum antibiotic prophylaxis group B streptococcal is recommended for the following:
1. Pregnant women with a positive screening culture unless a planned Cesarean section is performed in the absence of labor or rupture of membranes
2. Pregnant women who gave birth to a previous infant with invasive GBS disease
3. Pregnant women with documented GBS bacteriuria during the current pregnancy
4. Pregnant women whose culture status is unknown (culture not performed or result not available) and who also have delivery at <37 weeks of gestation, amniotic membrane rupture for ≥18 hours, or intrapartum temperature ≥100.4°F (≥38°C)
5. The recommended IAP regimen is penicillin G (5 million units IV initial dose, then 2.5 million units IV Q4h). In women with non-immediate-type penicillin-allergy, cefazolin (Ancef, 2 g initial dose, then 1 g Q8h) is recommended.

  D. Bed rest. Although bed rest is often prescribed for women at high risk for preterm labor and delivery, there are no conclusive studies documenting its benefit. A recent meta-analysis found no benefit to bed rest in the prevention of preterm labor or delivery.
References: See page 166.

Bleeding in the Second Half of Pregnancy

Bleeding in the second half of pregnancy occurs in 4% of all pregnancies. In 50% of cases, vaginal bleeding is secondary to placental abruption or placenta previa.

I. **Clinical evaluation of bleeding second half of pregnancy**
   A. **History** of trauma or pain and the amount and character of the bleeding should be assessed.
   B. **Physical examination**
      1. Vital signs and pulse pressure are measured. Hypotension and tachycardia are signs of serious hypovolemia.
      2. Fetal heart rate pattern and uterine activity are assessed.
      3. Ultrasound examination of the uterus, placenta and fetus should be completed.
      4. Speculum and digital pelvic examination should not be done until placenta previa has been excluded.
   C. **Laboratory Evaluation**
      1. **Hemoglobin** and hematocrit.
      2. **INR, partial thromboplastin time, platelet count, fibrinogen level, and fibrin split products** are checked when placental abruption is suspected or if there has been significant hemorrhage.
      3. **A red-top tube** of blood is used to perform a bedside clot test.
      4. **Blood type** and cross-match.
      5. **Urinalysis** for hematuria and proteinuria.
      6. The **Apt test** is used to distinguish maternal or fetal source of bleeding. (Vaginal blood is mixed with an equal part 0.25% sodium hydroxide. Fetal blood remains red; maternal blood turns brown.)
      7. **Kleihauer-Betke test** of maternal blood is used to quantify fetal to maternal hemorrhage.
II. **Placental abruption (abruptio placentae)** is defined as complete or partial placental separation from the decidua basalis after 20 weeks gestation.
   A. Placental abruption occurs in 1 in 100 deliveries.
   B. **Factors associated with placental abruption**
      1. Preeclampsia and hypertensive disorders
      2. History of placental abruption
      3. High multiparity
      4. Increasing maternal age
      5. Trauma
      6. Cigarette smoking
      7. Illicit drug use (especially cocaine)
      8. Excessive alcohol consumption
      9. Preterm premature rupture of the membranes
      10. Rapid uterine decompression after delivery of the first fetus in a twin gestation or rupture of membranes with polyhydramnios
      11. Uterine leiomyomas
   C. **Diagnosis of placental abruption**
      1. Abruption is characterized by vaginal bleeding, abdominal pain, uterine tenderness, and uterine contractions.
         a. Vaginal bleeding is visible in 80%; bleeding is concealed in 20%.
         b. Pain is usually of sudden onset, constant, and localized to the uterus and lower back.
         c. Localized or generalized uterine tenderness and increased uterine tone are found with severe placental abruption.

       d. An increase in uterine size may occur with placental abruption when the bleeding is concealed. Concealed bleeding may be detected by serial measurements of abdominal girth and fundal height.

       e. Amniotic fluid may be bloody.

       f. Fetal monitoring may detect distress.

       g. Placental abruption may cause preterm labor.

    2. **Uterine contractions** by tocodynamometry is the most sensitive indicator of abruption.

    3. **Laboratory findings** include proteinuria and a consumptive coagulopathy, characterized by decreased fibrinogen, prothrombin, factors V and VIII, and platelets. Fibrin split products are elevated.

    4. **Ultrasonography** has a sensitivity in detecting placental abruption of only 15%.

  D. **Management of placental abruption**

    1. **Mild placental abruption**

       a. If maternal stability and reassuring fetal surveillance are assured and the fetus is immature, close expectant observation with fetal monitoring is justified.

       b. Maternal hematologic parameters are monitored and abnormalities corrected.

       c. Tocolysis with magnesium sulfate is initiated if the fetus is immature.

    2. **Moderate to severe placental abruption**

       a. Shock is aggressively managed.

       b. **Coagulopathy**

         (1) Blood is transfused to replace blood loss.

         (2) Clotting factors may be replaced using cryoprecipitate or fresh-frozen plasma. One unit of fresh-frozen plasma increases fibrinogen by 10 mg/dL. Cryoprecipitate contains 250 mg fibrinogen/unit; 4 gm (15-20 U) is an effective dose.

         (3) Platelet transfusion is indicated if the platelet count is less than 50,000/mcL. One unit of platelets raises the platelet count 5000-10,000/mcL; 4 to 6 U is the smallest useful dose.

       c. **Oxygen** should be administered and urine output monitored with a Foley catheter.

       d. Vaginal delivery is expedited in all but the mildest cases once the mother has been stabilized. Amniotomy and oxytocin (Pitocin) augmentation may be used. Cesarean section is indicated for fetal distress, severe abruption, or failed trial of labor.

III. **Placenta previa** occurs when any part of the placenta implants in the lower uterine segment. It is associated with a risk of serious maternal hemorrhage. Placenta previa occurs in 1 in 200 pregnancies. Ninety percent of placenta previas diagnosed in the second trimester resolve spontaneously.

  A. **Total placenta previa** occurs when the internal cervical os is completely covered by placenta.

  B. **Partial placenta previa** occurs when part of the cervical os is covered by placenta.

  C. **Marginal placenta previa** occurs when the placental edge is located within 2 cm of the cervical os.

  D. **Clinical evaluation**

    1. Placenta previa presents with a sudden onset of painless vaginal bleeding in the second or third trimester. The peak incidence occurs at 34 weeks. The initial bleeding usually resolves spontaneously and then recurs later in pregnancy.

    2. One fourth of patients present with bleeding and uterine contractions.

  E. **Ultrasonography** is accurate in diagnosing placenta previa.

  F. **Management of placenta previa**

    1. In a pregnancy ≥36 weeks with documented fetal lung maturity, the neonate should be immediately delivered by cesarean section.

    2. Low vertical uterine incision is probably safer in patients with an anterior placenta. Incisions through the placenta should be avoided.

    3. If severe hemorrhage jeopardizes the mother or fetus, cesarean section is indicated regardless of gestational age.
    4. Expectant management is appropriate for immature fetuses if bleeding is not excessive, maternal physical activity can be restricted, intercourse and douching can be prohibited, and the hemoglobin can be maintained at ≥10 mg/dL.
    5. Rh immunoglobulin is administered to Rh-negative-unsensitized patients.
    6. Delivery is indicated once fetal lung maturity has been documented.
    7. Tocolysis with magnesium sulfate may be used for immature fetuses.

IV. Cervical bleeding
  A. Cytologic sampling is necessary.
  B. Bleeding can be controlled with cauterization or packing.
  C. Bacterial and viral cultures are sometimes diagnostic.

V. Cervical polyps
  A. Bleeding is usually self-limited.
  B. Trauma should be avoided.
  C. Polypectomy may control bleeding and yield a histologic diagnosis.

VI. Bloody show is a frequent benign cause of late third trimester bleeding. It is characterized by blood-tinged mucus associated with cervical change.

References: See page 166.

Preeclampsia-eclampsia and Chronic Hypertension

The are four major hypertensive disorders in pregnancy are preeclampsia-eclampsia, chronic hypertension, preeclampsia superimposed upon chronic hypertension, and gestational hypertension. Preeclampsia is characterized by hypertension and proteinuria developing after 20 weeks of gestation. Chronic hypertension is defined as systolic pressure ≥140 mm Hg, diastolic pressure ≥90 mm Hg, or both that antedates pregnancy or is present before the 20th week of pregnancy.

I. Incidence and risk factors for preeclampsia
  A. Hypertensive disorders occur in about 12 to 22 percent of pregnancies. Preeclampsia occurs in 3 to 8 percent of pregnancies. A woman under the age of 20 years who is undergoing her first pregnancy is at increased risk for preeclampsia. The primigravid state is a predisposing factor. The incidence of preeclampsia in a second pregnancy is less than 1 percent in women who have had a normotensive first pregnancy, as compared to 5-7 percent in women who had preeclampsia during the first pregnancy.
  B. Risk factors for preeclampsia:
    1. Primigravid state
    2. History of preeclampsia
    3. A higher blood pressure at the initiation of pregnancy and a large body size
    4. A family history of preeclampsia is associated with a two to fivefold increase in risk
    5. Multiple pregnancy
    6. Preexisting maternal hypertension
    7. Pregestational diabetes
    8. Antiphospholipid antibody syndrome
    9. Vascular or connective tissue disease
    10. Advanced maternal age (>35 to 40 years)

II. Clinical manifestations of preeclampsia
  A. Preeclampsia is characterized by the gradual development of hypertension, proteinuria, and edema in pregnancy, particularly in a primigravida. These findings typically become apparent in the latter part of the third trimester and progress until delivery. In some women, however, symptoms begin in the latter half of the second trimester. Signs and symptoms

of preeclampsia occurring before 20 weeks of gestation are unusual unless there is an underlying molar pregnancy, drug use or withdrawal, or chromosomal aneuploidy in the fetus.

B. **Hypertension.** Pregnancy related hypertension is defined as a systolic blood pressure greater than 140 mm Hg or diastolic blood pressure greater than 90 mm Hg in a woman who was normotensive prior to 20 weeks of gestation. Hypertension is usually the earliest clinical finding of preeclampsia. The blood pressure (BP) may rise in the second trimester, but usually does not reach the hypertensive range (>140/90) until the third trimester, often after the 37th week of gestation.

C. **Proteinuria.** In addition to hypertension, most patients also have proteinuria (ie, 1+ on dipstick or 0.3 g protein or greater in a 24-hour urine specimen).

D. **Eclampsia** refers to the development of grand mal seizures in a woman with preeclampsia. Preeclampsia-eclampsia is caused by generalized vasospasm, activation of the coagulation system, and changes in autoregulatory systems related to blood pressure control.

E. **Edema and intravascular volume.** Most women with preeclampsia have edema. Although peripheral edema is common in normal pregnancy, sudden and rapid weight gain and facial edema often occur in women who develop preeclampsia.

F. **Hematologic changes.** Increased platelet turnover is a consistent feature of preeclampsia. The most common coagulation abnormality in preeclampsia is thrombocytopenia.

G. **Liver involvement** may present as right upper quadrant or epigastric pain, elevated liver enzymes and subcapsular hemorrhage or hepatic rupture.

H. **Central nervous system.** Headache, blurred vision, scotomata, and, rarely, cortical blindness are manifestations of preeclampsia; seizures in a preeclamptic woman are defined as eclampsia.

I. **Fetus and placenta.** The fetal consequences are fetal growth restriction and oligohydramnios. Severe or early onset preeclampsia result in the greatest decrements in birth weight.

III. **Diagnosis**

A. The diagnosis of preeclampsia is largely based upon clinical features developing after 20 weeks of gestation in a woman who was previously normotensive.

Diagnosis of Preeclampsia

Systolic blood pressure greater than 140 mm Hg
or
Diastolic blood pressure greater than 90 mm Hg
AND
A random urine protein determination of 1+ on dipstick or 30 mg/dL or proteinuria of 0.3 g or greater in a 24-hour urine specimen

---

B. **Plasma uric acid concentration.** Preeclampsia is typically associated with a rise in the plasma urate level to above 5.5 to 6 mg/dL.

C. **Laboratory evaluation:**
   1. Hematocrit: hemoconcentration supports the diagnosis of preeclampsia
   2. Platelet count
   3. Quantification of protein excretion
   4. Serum creatinine concentration
   5. Serum uric acid concentration
   6. Serum alanine and aspartate aminotransferase concentrations (ALT, AST)
   7. Lactic acid dehydrogenase concentration (LDH) and red blood cell smear may indicate the presence of microangiopathic hemolysis.

Criteria for Severe Preeclampsia

New onset proteinuria hypertension and at least one of the following:
Symptoms of central nervous system dysfunction:
    Blurred vision, scotomata, altered mental status, severe headache
Symptoms of liver capsule distention:
    Right upper quadrant or epigastric pain
Hepatocellular injury
    Serum transaminase concentration at least twice normal
Severe blood pressure elevation:
    Systolic blood pressure ≥ 160 mm Hg or diastolic ≥ 110 mm Hg on two occasions at least six hours apart
Thrombocytopenia
    Less than 100,000 platelets per mm^3
Proteinuria:
    Over 5 grams in 24 hours or 3+ or more on two random samples four hours apart
Oliguria <500 mL in 24 hours
Intrauterine fetal growth restriction
Pulmonary edema or cyanosis
Cerebrovascular accident
Coagulopathy

IV. **Treatment of preeclampsia**
  A. The definitive treatment of preeclampsia is delivery. Delivery is recommended for women with mild preeclampsia at or near term and for most women with severe preeclampsia regardless of gestational age, except less than 33 weeks of gestation whose only criterion for severe disease is:
    1. Severe proteinuria (greater than 5 g in 24 hours).
    2. Mild intrauterine fetal growth restriction (fifth to tenth percentile).
    3. Severe preeclampsia by blood pressure criteria alone before 32 weeks of gestation, if there is blood pressure reduction and resolution of any laboratory abnormalities after hospitalization.
  B. **Treatment of hypertension.** Antihypertensive treatment is indicated if the systolic blood pressure is ≥ 170 mm Hg. The preferred agents are methyldopa for prolonged antenatal therapy, and hydralazine, labetalol or nifedipine for peripartum treatment of acute hypertensive episodes. Sodium restriction and diuretics have no role in therapy. Restricted physical activity can lower blood pressure.

Acute Treatment of Severe Hypertension in Preeclampsia

The goal is a gradual reduction of blood pressure to a level below 160/105 mm Hg. Sudden and severe hypotension should be avoided.

Hydralazine: 5 mg IV, repeat 5 to 10 mg IV every 20 minutes to maximum cumulative total of 20 mg or until blood pressure is controlled.

Labetalol (Trandate): 20 mg IV, followed by 40 mg, then 80 mg, then 80 mg at 10 minute intervals until the desired response is achieved or a maximum total dose of 220 mg is administered.

Methyldopa (Aldomet) 250 mg BID orally, maximum dose 4 g/day

Fetal Assessment in Preeclampsia	
Mild preeclampsia	Daily fetal movement counting Ultrasound examination for estimation of fetal weight and amniotic fluid determination at diagnosis. Repeat in three weeks if the initial examination is normal, twice weekly if there is evidence of fetal growth restriction or oligohydramnios. Nonstress test and/or biophysical profile once or twice weekly. Testing should be repeated immediately if there is an abrupt change in maternal condition.
Severe preeclampsia	Daily nonstress testing and/or biophysical profile

C. **Antenatal corticosteroids** to promote fetal lung maturation should be administered to women less than 34 weeks of gestation who are at high risk for delivery within the next seven days. Betamethasone (two doses of 12 mg given intramuscularly 24 hours apart) or dexamethasone (four doses of 6 mg given intramuscularly 12 hours apart) may be used.

D. **Maternal monitoring.** Laboratory evaluation (eg, hematocrit, platelet count, creatinine, urine protein, LDH, AST, ALT, uric acid) should be repeated once or twice weekly in women with mild stable preeclampsia.

E. **Women with severe preeclampsia** should be delivered or hospitalized for the duration of pregnancy. Prolonged antepartum management may be considered in selected women under 32 weeks of gestation, such as those whose condition improves after hospitalization and who have no evidence of end-organ dysfunction or fetal deterioration.

F. **Timing and indications for delivery**. Delivery at or by 40 weeks of gestation should be considered for all women with preeclampsia. Women with mild disease and a favorable cervix may benefit from induction as early as 38 weeks, while those with stable severe disease should be delivered after 32 to 34 weeks if possible (with demonstration of fetal pulmonary maturity).

Indications for Delivery in Preeclampsia	
Maternal indications	Gestational age greater than or equal to 38 weeks of gestation Platelet count less than 100,000 cells per mm^3 Deteriorating liver function Progressive deterioration in renal function Abruptio placentae Persistent severe headaches or visual changes Persistent severe epigastric pain, nausea, or vomiting
Fetal indications	Severe fetal growth restriction Nonreassuring results from fetal testing Oligohydramnios

G. **Route of delivery.** Delivery is usually by the vaginal route, with cesarean delivery reserved for obstetrical indications. Cervical ripening agents may be used if the cervix is not favorable.

H. **Anticonvulsant therapy**
1. Anticonvulsant therapy is initiated during labor until 24 to 48 hours postpartum. Magnesium sulfate is the drug of choice for seizure prevention.
2. **Magnesium regimen.** A loading dose of 6 g intravenously is given, followed by 2 g/h as a continuous infusion.

    I. **Postpartum course.** Hypertension due to preeclampsia resolves postpartum, often within a few days, but sometimes takes a few weeks.

V. Management of eclampsia

    A. Maintenance of airway patency and prevention of aspiration are the initial management priorities. The patient should be rolled onto her left side and a padded tongue blade placed in her mouth, if possible.

    B. **Control of convulsions.** Magnesium sulfate, 2 to 4 g IV push repeated every 15 minutes to a maximum of 6 g. **Maintenance dose of magnesium sulfate:** 2 to 3 g/hour by continuous intravenous infusion. Diazepam may also be given as 5 mg IV push repeated as needed to a maximum cumulative dose of 20 mg to stop the convulsions; however, benzodiazepines have profound depressant effects on the fetus.

VI. Preexistent hypertension

    A. Methyldopa (Aldomet) has been most widely used and long-term safety to the fetus has been clearly demonstrated. ACE inhibitors should not be continued in pregnancy. ß-blockers are generally safe, although they may impair fetal growth when used early in pregnancy, particularly atenolol. Thiazide diuretics can be continued as long as volume depletion is avoided.

Treatment of Hypertension in Pregnancy	
Drug	**Dose**
Methyldopa (Aldomet)	250 mg BID orally, maximum dose 4 g/day
Labetalol (Trandate)	100 mg BID orally, maximum dose 2400 mg/day

    B. **Risks of chronic hypertension.** Chronic hypertension is associated with a threefold increase in perinatal mortality, a twofold increase in abruptio placentae, and an increased rate of impaired fetal growth. There is also a higher rate of preterm delivery before 35 weeks of gestation.

    C. **Indications for treatment**. Indications for antihypertensive therapy are a diastolic pressure persistently above 100 mm Hg, systolic pressure ≥150 to 180 mm Hg or signs of hypertensive end-organ damage. Severe hypertension (blood pressure of 180/110 mmHg or higher) requires intravenous therapy. Hydralazine and labetalol are the drugs of choice for intravenous administration.

    D. **Fetal surveillance** is warranted when there is preeclampsia or intrauterine growth restriction. Serial sonographic assessment of fetal growth is indicated, with nonstress testing or biophysical profile examination weekly starting at 28 weeks, increasing to twice-weekly at 32 weeks.

    E. **Delivery.** Woman with mild, uncomplicated chronic hypertension can be allowed to go into spontaneous labor and deliver at term. Earlier delivery can be considered for women with superimposed preeclampsia or pregnancy complications (eg, fetal growth restriction, previous stillbirth).

References: See page 166.

Herpes Simplex Virus Infections in Pregnancy

Herpes simplex virus (HSV) type 2 is primarily responsible for genital HSV disease. Maternal-fetal transmission of HSV is the major consequence of maternal HSV infection, resulting in encephalitis, disseminated disease, and skin disease. The most common mode of transmission is via contact of the fetus with infected vaginal secretions during delivery.

I. **Diagnosis**
   A. **Risk factors.** Black or Hispanic race, age, and years of sexual experience are highly correlated with HSV-2 infection. Other factors include lower family income, lower level of education, multiple sexual partners, and having other sexually transmitted diseases.
   B. The gold standard for diagnosis of acute HSV infection is viral culture, which may become positive within two to three days after inoculation.
   C. Polymerase chain reaction (PCR) is used to rapidly detect HSV DNA from lesions or genital secretions and is superior to other tests. PCR has been used to detect HSV from pregnant women with recurrent HSV at delivery and their infants in instances in which HSV cultures were negative.

II. **Clinical presentation**
   A. **Primary genital episode genital HSV** is characterized by multiple painful vesicles in clusters. They may be associated with pruritus, dysuria, vaginal discharge, and tender regional adenopathy. Fever, malaise, and myalgia often occur one to two days prior to the appearance of lesions. The lesions may last four to five days prior to crusting. The skin will reepithelialize in about 10 days. Viral shedding may last for 10 to 12 days after reepithelialization.
   B. **Nonprimary first-episode genital HSV** refers to patients with preexisting antibodies to one of the two types of virus who acquire the other virus and develop genital lesions. Nonprimary disease is less severe with fewer systemic symptoms, and less local pain.
   C. **Recurrent HSV episodes** are characterized by local pain or paresthesia followed by vesicular lesions. They are generally fewer in number and often unilateral but may be painful.

III. **Pregnancy**
   A. **Estimated risks of maternal-fetal transmission:**
      1. Primary or nonprimary first episode with an active lesion at delivery: 50 percent
      2. Asymptomatic first episode: 33 percent
      3. Recurrent HSV with active lesion: 3 to 4 percent
      4. **Asymptomatic recurrence:** 0.04 percent

IV. **Neonatal effects**
   A. HSV neonatal infection is most often acquired through the birth canal. The incidence of neonatal HSV infection is 1 in 3000. Approximately 60 to 70 percent of infected neonates are infected with HSV-2.
   B. The **categories of neonatal disease** include localized disease of the skin, eyes and mouth (SEM), central nervous system (CNS) disease with or without SEM involvement, and disseminated disease
   C. The mortality rate is 15 percent among children with CNS disease and 57 percent with disseminated disease.

V. **Treatment**
   A. **Primary infection**
      1. Acyclovir (Zovirax) therapy (200 mg PO five times per day or 400 mg PO TID for 7 to 14 days) and analgesia is recommended. Acyclovir is safe in pregnancy. Acyclovir reduces the duration of viral shedding.
      2. Suppressive therapy (400 mg PO BID) for the remainder of pregnancy should usually be administered because acyclovir may prevent symptomatic HSV recurrences at term.
   B. **Recurrent infection.** Acyclovir reduces shedding by 80 percent and may reduce clinical recurrences. Women with frequent HSV recurrences may benefit from suppression (acyclovir 400 mg PO BID) near term.
   C. **Role of cesarean section**
      1. Cesarean section should be offered to women who have active lesions or symptoms of vulvar pain or burning at the time of delivery and a history of genital herpes.
      2. Prophylactic cesarean section is not recommended for women with recurrent HSV and no evidence of active lesions at the time of delivery. Lesions which have crusted fully are considered healed and not active.

3. Cesarean section is not recommended for women with recurrent genital herpes and active nongenital HSV lesions. The lesions should be covered with an occlusive dressing.
   - **D. Very preterm infants (<30 to 32 weeks) in preterm labor:** If the mother has active HSV, delay of delivery for betamethasone therapy is appropriate. Cesarean section after either documented pulmonary maturity or betamethasone would be appropriate if active lesions are present. The use of acyclovir during this time may be helpful to shorten the time of active lesions for the mother.
   - E. Herpes cultures or the more sensitive PCR test is often performed on the neonate at delivery to identify exposed infants.

References: See page 166.

Dystocia and Augmentation of Labor

I. Normal labor
A. First stage of labor
1. The first stage of labor consists of the period from the onset of labor until complete cervical dilation (10 cm). This stage is divided into the latent phase and the active phase.
2. **Latent phase**
   - a. During the latent phase, uterine contractions are infrequent and irregular and result in only modest discomfort. They result in gradual effacement and dilation of the cervix.
   - b. A prolonged latent phase is one that exceeds 20 hours in the nullipara or one that exceeds 14 hours in the multipara.
3. **Active phase**
   - a. The active phase of labor occurs when the cervix reaches 3-4 cm of dilatation.
   - b. The active phase of labor is characterized by an increased rate of cervical dilation and by descent of the presenting fetal part.

B. Second stage of labor
1. **The second stage of labor** consists of the period from complete cervical dilation (10 cm) until delivery of the infant. This stage is usually brief, averaging 20 minutes for parous women and 50 minutes for nulliparous women.
2. The duration of the second stage of labor is unrelated to perinatal outcome in the absence of a nonreassuring fetal heart rate pattern as long as progress occurs.

II. Abnormal labor
A. **Dystocia** is defined as difficult labor or childbirth resulting from abnormalities of the cervix and uterus, the fetus, the maternal pelvis, or a combination of these factors.
B. **Cephalopelvic disproportion** is a disparity between the size of the maternal pelvis and the fetal head that precludes vaginal delivery. This condition can rarely be diagnosed in advance.
C. **Slower-than-normal (protraction disorders) or complete cessation of progress (arrest disorder)** are disorders that can be diagnosed only after the parturient has entered the active phase of labor.

III. Assessment of labor abnormalities
A. **Labor abnormalities caused by inadequate uterine contractility (powers).** The minimal uterine contractile pattern of women in spontaneous labor consists of 3 to 5 contractions in a 10-minute period.
B. **Labor abnormalities caused by fetal characteristics (passenger)**
1. Assessment of the fetus consists of estimating fetal weight and position. Estimations of fetal size, even those obtained by ultrasonography, are frequently inaccurate.
2. In the first stage of labor, the diagnosis of dystocia can not be made unless the active phase of labor and adequate uterine contractile forces have been present.

3. Fetal anomalies such as hydrocephaly, encephalocele, and soft tissue tumors may obstruct labor. Fetal imaging should be considered when malpresentation or anomalies are suspected based on vaginal or abdominal examination or when the presenting fetal part is persistently high.

C. **Labor abnormalities due to the pelvic passage (passage)**
   1. Inefficient uterine action should be corrected before attributing dystocia to a pelvic problem.
   2. The bony pelvis is very rarely the factor that limits vaginal delivery of a fetus in cephalic presentation. Radiographic pelvimetry is of limited value in managing most cephalic presentations.
   3. Clinical pelvimetry can only be useful to qualitatively identify the general architectural features of the pelvis.

IV. **Augmentation of labor**
   A. Uterine hypocontractility should be augmented only after both the maternal pelvis and fetal presentation have been assessed.
   B. Contraindications to augmentation include placenta or vasa previa, umbilical cord prolapse, prior classical uterine incision, pelvic structural deformities, and invasive cervical cancer.
   C. **Oxytocin (Pitocin)**
      1. The goal of oxytocin administration is to stimulate uterine activity that is sufficient to produce cervical change and fetal descent while avoiding uterine hyperstimulation and fetal compromise.
      2. **Minimally effective uterine activity** is 3 contractions per 10 minutes averaging greater than 25 mm Hg above baseline. A maximum of 5 contractions in a 10-minute period with resultant cervical dilatation is considered adequate.
      3. **Hyperstimulation** is characterized by more than five contractions in 10 minutes, contractions lasting 2 minutes or more, or contractions of normal duration occurring within 1 minute of each other.
      4. Oxytocin is administered when a patient is progressing slowly through the latent phase of labor or has a protraction or an arrest disorder of labor, or when a hypotonic uterine contraction pattern is identified.
      5. A pelvic examination should be performed before initiation of oxytocin infusion.
      6. Oxytocin is usually diluted 10 units in 1 liter of normal saline IVPB.

Labor Stimulation with Oxytocin (Pitocin)			
Starting Dose (mU/min)	**Incremental Increase (mU/min)**	**Dosage Interval (min)**	**Maximum Dose (mU/min)**
6	6	15	40

   7. **Management of oxytocin-induced hyperstimulation**
      a. The most common adverse effect of hyperstimulation is fetal heart rate deceleration associated with uterine hyperstimulation. Stopping or decreasing the dose of oxytocin may correct the abnormal pattern.
      b. Additional measures may include changing the patient to the lateral decubitus position and administering oxygen or more intravenous fluid.
      c. If oxytocin-induced uterine hyperstimulation does not respond to conservative measures, intravenous terbutaline (0.125-0.25 mg) or magnesium sulfate (2-6 g in 10-20% dilution) may be used to stop uterine contractions.

References: See page 166.

Fetal Macrosomia

Excessive birth weight is associated with an increased risk of maternal and neonatal injury. Macrosomia is defined as a fetus with an estimated weight of more than 4,500 grams, regardless of gestational age.

I. **Diagnosis of macrosomia**
   A. Clinical estimates of fetal weight based on Leopold's maneuvers or fundal height measurements are often inaccurate.
   B. Diagnosis of macrosomia requires ultrasound evaluation; however, estimation of fetal weight based on ultrasound is associated with a large margin of error.
   C. Maternal weight, height, previous obstetric history, fundal height, and the presence of gestational diabetes should be evaluated.

II. **Factors influencing fetal weight**
   A. **Gestational age.** Post-term pregnancy is a risk factor for macrosomia. At 42 weeks and beyond, 2.5% of fetuses weigh more than 4,500 g. Ten to twenty percent of macrosomic infants are post-term fetuses.
   B. **Maternal weight.** Heavy women have a greater risk of giving birth to excessively large infants. Fifteen to 35% of women who deliver macrosomic fetuses weigh 90 kg or more.
   C. **Multiparity.** Macrosomic infants are 2-3 times more likely to be born to parous women.
   D. **Macrosomia in a prior infant.** The risk of delivering an infant weighing more than 4,500 g is increased if a prior infant weighed more than 4,000 g.
   E. **Maternal diabetes**
      1. Maternal diabetes increases the risk of fetal macrosomia and shoulder dystocia.
      2. Cesarean delivery is indicated when the estimated fetal weight exceeds 4,500 g.

III. **Morbidity and mortality**
   A. **Abnormalities of labor.** Macrosomic fetuses have a higher incidence of labor abnormalities and instrumental deliveries.
   B. **Maternal morbidity.** Macrosomic fetuses have a two- to threefold increased rate of cesarean delivery.
   C. **Birth injury**
      1. The incidence of birth injuries occurring during delivery of a macrosomic infant is much greater with vaginal than with cesarean birth. The most common injury is brachial plexus palsy, often caused by shoulder dystocia.
      2. The incidence of shoulder dystocia in infants weighing more than 4,500 g is 8-20%. Macrosomic infants also may sustain fractures of the clavicle or humerus.

IV. **Management of delivery**
   A. If the estimated fetal weight is greater than 4500 gm in the nondiabetic or greater than 4000 gm in the diabetic patient, delivery by cesarean section is indicated.
   B. **Management of shoulder dystocia**
      1. If a shoulder dystocia occurs, an assistant should provide suprapubic pressure to dislodge the impacted anterior fetal shoulder from the symphysis. McRoberts maneuver (extreme hip flexion) should be done simultaneously.
      2. If the shoulder remains impacted anteriorly, an ample episiotomy should be cut and the posterior arm delivered.
      3. In almost all instances, one or both of these procedures will result in successful delivery. The Zavanelli maneuver consists of replacement of the fetal lead into the vaginal canal and delivery by emergency cesarean section.
      4. Fundal pressure is not recommended because it often results in further impaction of the shoulder against the symphysis.

References: See page 166.

Shoulder Dystocia

Shoulder dystocia, defined as failure of the shoulders to deliver following the head, is an obstetric emergency. The incidence varies from 0.6% to 1.4% of all vaginal deliveries. Up to 30% of shoulder dystocias can result in brachial plexus injury; many fewer sustain serious asphyxia or death. Most commonly, size discrepancy secondary to fetal macrosomia is associated with difficult shoulder delivery. Causal factors of macrosomia include maternal diabetes, postdates gestation, and obesity. The fetus of the diabetic gravida may also have disproportionately large shoulders and body size compared with the head.

I. Prediction

A. The diagnosis of shoulder dystocia is made after delivery of the head. The "turtle" sign is the retraction of the chin against the perineum or retraction of the head into the birth canal. This sign demonstrates that the shoulder girdle is resisting entry into the pelvic inlet, and possibly impaction of the anterior shoulder.

B. Macrosomia has the strongest association. ACOG defines macrosomia as an estimated fetal weight (EFW) greater than 4500 g.

C. Risk factors for macrosomia include maternal birth weight, prior macrosomia, preexisting diabetes, obesity, multiparity, advanced maternal age, and a prior shoulder dystocia. The recurrence rate has been reported to be 13.8%, nearly seven times the primary rate. Shoulder dystocia occurs in 5.1% of obese women. In the antepartum period, risk factors include gestational diabetes, excessive weight gain, short stature, macrosomia, and postterm pregnancy. Intrapartum factors include prolonged second stage of labor, abnormal first stage, arrest disorders, and instrumental (especially midforceps) delivery. Many shoulder dystocias will occur in the absence of any risk factors.

II. Management

A. Shoulder dystocia is a medical and possibly surgical emergency. Two assistants should be called for if not already present, as well as an anesthesiologist and pediatrician. A generous episiotomy should be cut. The following sequence is suggested:

1. **McRoberts maneuver:** The legs are removed from the lithotomy position and flexed at the hips, with flexion of the knees against the abdomen. Two assistants are required. This maneuver may be performed prophylactically in anticipation of a difficult delivery.

2. **Suprapubic pressure:** An assistant is requested to apply pressure downward, above the symphysis pubis. This can be done in a lateral direction to help dislodge the anterior shoulder from behind the pubic symphysis. It can also be performed in anticipation of a difficult delivery. Fundal pressure may increase the likelihood of uterine rupture and is contraindicated.

3. **Rotational maneuvers:** The Woods' corkscrew maneuver consists of placing two fingers against the anterior aspect of the posterior shoulder. Gentle upward rotational pressure is applied so that the posterior shoulder girdle rotates anteriorly, allowing it to be delivered first. The Rubin maneuver is the reverse of Woods's maneuver. Two fingers are placed against the posterior aspect of the posterior (or anterior) shoulder and forward pressure applied. This results in adduction of the shoulders and displacement of the anterior shoulder from behind the symphysis pubis.

4. **Posterior arm release:** The operator places a hand into the posterior vagina along the infant's back. The posterior arm is identified and followed to the elbow. The elbow is then swept across the chest, keeping the elbow flexed. The fetal forearm or hand is then grasped and the posterior arm delivered, followed by the anterior shoulder. If

the fetus still remains undelivered, vaginal delivery should be abandoned and the Zavanelli maneuver performed followed by cesarean delivery.

5. **Zavanelli maneuver:** The fetal head is replaced into the womb. Tocolysis is recommended to produce uterine relaxation. The maneuver consists of rotation of the head to occiput anterior. The head is then flexed and pushed back into the vagina, followed abdominal delivery. Immediate preparations should be made for cesarean delivery.

6. If cephalic replacement fails, an emergency symphysiotomy should be performed. The urethra should be laterally displaced to minimize the risk of lower urinary tract injury.

B. The McRoberts maneuver alone will successfully alleviate the shoulder dystocia in 42% to 79% of cases. For those requiring additional maneuvers, vaginal delivery can be expected in more than 90%. Finally, favorable results have been reported for the Zavanelli maneuver in up to 90%.

References: See page 166.

Postdates Pregnancy

A term gestation is defined as one completed in 38 to 42 weeks. Pregnancy is considered prolonged or postdates when it exceeds 294 days or 42 weeks from the first day of the last menstrual period (LMP). About 10% of those pregnancies are postdates. The incidence of patients reaching the 42nd week is 3-12%.

I. **Morbidity and mortality**
   A. The rate of maternal, fetal, and neonatal complications increases with gestational age. The cesarean delivery rate more than doubles when passing the 42nd week compared with 40 weeks because of cephalopelvic disproportion resulting from larger infants and by fetal intolerance of labor.
   B. Neonatal complications from postdates pregnancies include placental insufficiency, birth trauma from macrosomia, meconium aspiration syndrome, and oligohydramnios.

II. **Diagnosis**
   A. The accurate diagnosis of postdates pregnancy can be made only by proper dating. The estimated date of confinement (EDC) is most accurately determined early in pregnancy. An EDC can be calculated by subtracting 3 months from the first day of the last menses and adding 7 days (Naegele's rule). Other clinical parameters that should be consistent with the EDC include maternal perception of fetal movements (quickening) at about 16 to 20 weeks; first auscultation of fetal heart tones with Doppler ultrasound by 12 weeks; uterine size at early examination (first trimester) consistent with dates; and, at 20 weeks, a fundal height 20 cm above the symphysis pubis or at the umbilicus.

Clinical Estimates of Gestational Age	
Parameter	**Gestational age (weeks)**
Positive urine hCG	5
Fetal heart tones by Doppler	11 to 12

Quickening
    Primigravida
    Multigravida
	
	20
	16

Parameter	Gestational age (weeks)
Fundal height at umbilicus	20

  B. In patients without reliable clinical data, ultrasound is beneficial. Ultrasonography is most accurate in early gestation. The crown-rump length becomes less accurate after 12 weeks in determining gestational age because the fetus begins to curve.

III. Management of the postdates pregnancy

  A. A postdates patient with a favorable cervix should receive induction of labor. Only 8.2% of pregnancies at 42 weeks have a ripe cervix (Bishop score >6). Induction at 41 weeks with PGE_2 cervical ripening lowers the cesarean delivery rate.

  B. **Cervical ripening with prostaglandin**
    1. Prostaglandin E_2 gel is a valuable tool for improving cervical ripeness and for increasing the likelihood of successful induction.
    2. Pre- and postapplication fetal monitoring are usually utilized. If the fetus has a nonreassuring heart rate tracing or there is excessive uterine activity, the use of PGE_2 gel is not advisable. The incidence of uterine hyperstimulation with PGE_2 gel, at approximately 5%, is comparable to that seen with oxytocin. Current PGE_2 modalities include the following:
      a. 2 to 3 mg of PGE_2 suspended in a gel placed intravaginally
      b. 0.5 mg of PGE_2 suspended in a gel placed intracervically (Prepidil)
      c. 10 mg of PGE_2 gel in a sustained-release tape (Cervidil)
      d. 25 µg of PGE_1 (one-fourth of tablet) placed intravaginally every 3 to 4 hours (misoprostol)

  C. **Stripping of membranes**, starting at 38 weeks and repeated weekly may be an effective method of inducing labor in post-term women with a favorable cervix. Stripping of membranes is performed by placing a finger in the cervical os and circling 3 times in the plane between the fetal head and cervix.

  D. **Expectant management with antenatal surveillance**
    1. Begin testing near the end of the 41st week of pregnancy. Antepartum testing consists of the nonstress test (NST) combined with the amniotic fluid index (AFI) twice weekly. The false-negative rate is 6.1/1000 (stillbirth within 1 week of a reassuring test) with twice weekly NSTs.
    2. The AFI involves measuring the deepest vertical fluid pocket in each uterine quadrant and summing the four together. Less than 5 cm is considered oligohydramnios, 5 to 8 cm borderline, and greater than 8 cm normal.

  E. **Fetal movement counting (kick counts).** Fetal movement has been correlated with fetal health. It consist of having the mother lie on her side and count fetal movements. Perception of 10 distinct movements in a period of up to 2 hours is considered reassuring. After 10 movements have been perceived, the count may be discontinued.

  F. **Delivery** is indicated if the amniotic fluid index is less than 5 cm, a nonreactive non-stress test is identified, or if decelerations are identified on the nonstress test.

  G. **Intrapartum management**
    1. **Meconium staining** is more common in postdates pregnancies. If oligohydramnios is present, amnioinfusion dilutes meconium and decreases the number of infants with meconium below the vocal cords. Instillation of normal saline through an intrauterine pressure catheter may reduce variable decelerations.
    2. **Macrosomia** should be suspected in all postdates gestations. Fetal weight should be estimated prior to labor in all postdates pregnancies. Ultrasonographic weight predictions generally fall within 20% of the actual birth weight.

3. **Management of suspected macrosomia.** The pediatrician and anesthesiologist should be notified so that they can prepare for delivery. Cesarean delivery should be considered in patients with an estimated fetal weight greater than 4500 g and a marginal pelvis, or someone with a previous difficult vaginal delivery with a similarly sized or larger infant.
4. Intrapartum asphyxia is also more common in the postdates pregnancy. Therefore, close observation of the fetal heart rate tracing is necessary during labor. Variable decelerations representing cord compression are frequently seen in postdates pregnancies
5. Cord compression can be treated with amnioinfusion, which can reduce variable decelerations. Late decelerations are more direct evidence of fetal hypoxia. If intermittent, late decelerations are managed conservatively with positioning and oxygen. If persistent late decelerations are associated with decreased variability or an elevated baseline fetal heart rate, immediate evaluation or delivery is indicated. This additional evaluation can include observation for fetal heart acceleration following fetal scalp or acoustic stimulation, or a fetal scalp pH.

References: See page 166.

Induction of Labor

Induction of labor refers to stimulation of uterine contractions prior to the onset of spontaneous labor. Between 1990 and 1998, the rate of labor induction doubled from 10 to 20 percent.

I. **Indications for labor induction:**
   A. Preeclampsia/eclampsia, and other hypertensive diseases
   B. Maternal diabetes mellitus
   C. Prelabor rupture of membranes
   D. Chorioamnionitis
   E. Intrauterine fetal growth restriction (IUGR)
   F. Isoimmunization
   G. In-utero fetal demise
   H. Postterm pregnancy
II. **Absolute contraindications to labor induction:**
   A. Prior classical uterine incision
   B. Active genital herpes infection
   C. Placenta or vasa previa
   D. Umbilical cord prolapse
   E. Fetal malpresentation, such as transverse lie
II. **Requirements for induction**
   A. Prior to undertaking labor induction, assessments of gestational age, fetal size and presentation, clinical pelvimetry, and cervical examination should be performed. Fetal maturity should be evaluated, and amniocentesis for fetal lung maturity may be needed prior to induction.
   B. **Clinical criteria that confirm term gestation:**
      1. Fetal heart tones documented for 30 weeks by Doppler.
      2. Thirty-six weeks have elapsed since a serum or urine human chorionic gonadotropin (hCG) pregnancy test was positive.
      3. Ultrasound measurement of the crown-rump length at 6 to 11 weeks of gestation or biparietal diameter/femur length at 12 to 20 weeks of gestation support a clinically determined gestational age equal to or greater than 39 weeks.
   C. **Assessment of cervical ripeness**
      1. A cervical examination should be performed before initiating attempts at labor induction.

2. The modified Bishop scoring system is most commonly used to assess the cervix. A score is calculated based upon the station of the presenting part and cervical dilatation, effacement, consistency, and position.

Modified Bishop Scoring System				
	0	1	2	3
Dilation, cm	Closed	1-2	3-4	5-6
Effacement, percent	0-30	40-50	60-70	≥80
Station*	-3	-2	-1, 0	+1, +2
Cervical consistency	Firm	Medium	Soft	
Position of the cervix	Posterior	Midposition	Anterior	
* Based on a -3 to +3 scale.				

3. The likelihood of a vaginal delivery after labor induction is similar to that after spontaneous onset of labor if the Bishop score is ≥8.

III. Induction of labor with oxytocin
   A. The uterine response to exogenous oxytocin administration is periodic uterine contractions.
   B. Oxytocin regimen (Pitocin)
      1. Oxytocin is given intravenously. Oxytocin is diluted by placing 10 units in 1000 mL of normal saline, yielding an oxytocin concentration of 10 mU/mL. Begin at 6 mU/min and increase by 6 mU/min every 15 minutes.
      2. Active management of labor regimens use a high-dose oxytocin infusion with short incremental time intervals.

High Dose Oxytocin Regimen

Begin oxytocin 6 mU per minute intravenously
Increase dose by 6 mU per minute every 15 minutes
Maximum dose: 40 mU per minute
Maximum total dose administered-during-labor: 10 U Maximum duration of administration: six hours

3. The dose of maximum oxytocin is usually 40 mU/min. The dose is typically increased until contractions occur at two to three minute intervals.

IV. Cervical ripening agents
   A. A ripening process should be considered prior to use of oxytocin use when the cervix is unfavorable.
   B. Mechanical methods
      1. **Membrane stripping** is a widely utilized technique, which causes release of either prostaglandin F2-alpha from the decidua and adjacent membranes or prostaglandin E2 from the cervix. Weekly membrane stripping beginning at 38 weeks of gestation results in delivery within a shorter period of time (8.6 versus 15 days).
      2. **Amniotomy** is an effective method of labor induction when performed in women with partially dilated and effaced cervices. Caution should be exercised to ensure that the fetal vertex is well-applied to the cervix and the umbilical cord or other fetal part is not presenting.

    3. **Foley catheter.** An uninflated Foley catheter can be passed through an undilated cervix and then inflated. This technique is as effective as prostaglandin E2 gel. The use of extra-amniotic saline infusion with a balloon catheter or a double balloon catheter (Atad ripener) also appears to be effective for cervical ripening.

C. **Prostaglandins**
    1. Local administration of prostaglandins to the vagina or the endocervix is the route of choice because of fewer side effects and acceptable clinical response. Uncommon side effects include fever, chills, vomiting, and diarrhea.
    2. **Prepidil** contains 0.5 mg of dinoprostone in 2.5 mL of gel for intracervical administration. The dose can be repeated in 6 to 12 hours if there is inadequate cervical change and minimal uterine activity following the first dose. The maximum cumulative dose is 1.5 mg (ie, 3 doses) within a 24-hour period. The time interval between the final dose and initiation of oxytocin should be 6 to 12 hours because of the potential for uterine hyperstimulation with concurrent oxytocin and prostaglandin administration.
    3. **Cervidil** is a vaginal insert containing 10 mg of dinoprostone in a timed-release formulation. The vaginal insert administers the medication at 0.3 mg/h and should be left in place for 12 hours. Oxytocin may be initiated 30 to 60 minutes after removal of the insert.
    4. An advantage of the vaginal insert over the gel formulation is that the insert can be removed in cases of uterine hyperstimulation or abnormalities of the fetal heart rate tracing.

V. **Complications of labor induction**
  A. **Hyperstimulation and tachysystole** may occur with use of prostaglandin compounds or oxytocin. Hyperstimulation is defined as uterine contractions lasting at least two minutes or five or more uterine contractions in 10 minutes. Tachysystole is defined as six or more contractions in 20 minutes.
  B. **Prostaglandin E2 (PGE2) preparations** have up to a 5 percent rate of uterine hyperstimulation. Fetal heart rate abnormalities can occur, but usually resolve upon removal of the drug. Rarely hyperstimulation or tachysystole can cause uterine rupture. Removing the PGE2 vaginal insert will usually help reverse the effects of the hyperstimulation and tachysystole. Cervical and vaginal lavage after local application of prostaglandin compounds is not helpful.
  C. If oxytocin is being infused, it should be discontinued to achieve a reassuring fetal heart rate pattern. Placing the woman in the left lateral position, administering oxygen, and increasing intravenous fluids may also be of benefit. Terbutaline 0.25 mg subcutaneously (a tocolytic) may be given.

References: See page 166.

Postpartum Hemorrhage

Obstetric hemorrhage remains a leading causes of maternal mortality. Postpartum hemorrhage is defined as the loss of more than 500 mL of blood following delivery. However, the average blood loss in an uncomplicated vaginal delivery is about 500 mL, with 5% losing more than 1,000 mL.

I. **Clinical evaluation of postpartum hemorrhage**
  A. **Uterine atony** is the most common cause of postpartum hemorrhage. Conditions associated with uterine atony include an overdistended uterus (eg, polyhydramnios, multiple gestation), rapid or prolonged labor, macrosomia, high parity, and chorioamnionitis.
  B. **Conditions associated with bleeding from trauma** include forceps delivery, macrosomia, precipitous labor and delivery, and episiotomy.
  C. **Conditions associated with bleeding from coagulopathy and thrombocytopenia** include abruptio placentae, amniotic fluid embolism, preeclampsia, coagulation disorders, autoimmune thrombocytopenia, and

anticoagulants.

D. **Uterine rupture** is associated with previous uterine surgery, internal podalic version, breech extraction, multiple gestation, and abnormal fetal presentation. High parity is a risk factor for both uterine atony and rupture.

E. **Uterine inversion** is detected by abdominal vaginal examination, which will reveal a uterus with an unusual shape after delivery.

II. **Management of postpartum hemorrhage**

A. **Following delivery** of the placenta, the uterus should be palpated to determine whether atony is present. If atony is present, vigorous fundal massage should be administered. If bleeding continues despite uterine massage, it can often be controlled with bimanual uterine compression.

B. **Genital tract lacerations** should be suspected in patients who have a firm uterus, but who continue to bleed. The cervix and vagina should be inspected to rule out lacerations. If no laceration is found but bleeding is still profuse, the uterus should be manually examined to exclude rupture.

C. **The placenta and uterus should be examined** for retained placental fragments. Placenta accreta is usually manifest by failure of spontaneous placental separation.

D. **Bleeding from non-genital areas** (venous puncture sites) suggests coagulopathy. Laboratory tests that confirm coagulopathy include INR, partial thromboplastin time, platelet count, fibrinogen, fibrin split products, and a clot retraction test.

E. **Medical management of postpartum hemorrhage**

1. **Oxytocin (Pitocin)** is usually given routinely immediately after delivery to stimulate uterine firmness and diminish blood loss. 20 units of oxytocin in 1,000 mL of normal saline or Ringer's lactate is administered at 100 drops/minute. Oxytocin should not be given as a rapid bolus injection because of the potential for circulatory collapse.

2. **Methylergonovine (Methergine)** 0.2 mg can be given IM if uterine massage and oxytocin are not effective in correcting uterine atony and provided there is no hypertension.

3. **15-methyl prostaglandin F2-alpha (Hemabate)**, one ampule (0.25 mg), can be given IM, with repeat injections every 20min, up to 4 doses can be given if hypertension is present; it is contraindicated in asthma.

Treatment of Postpartum Hemorrhage Secondary to Uterine Atony	
Drug	**Protocol**
Oxytocin	20 U in 1,000 mL of lactated Ringer's as IV infusion
Methylergonovine (Methergine)	0.2 mg IM
Prostaglandin (15 methyl PGF2-alpha [Hemabate, Prostin/15M])	0.25 mg as IM every 15-60 minutes as necessary

F. **Volume replacement**

1. Patients with postpartum hemorrhage that is refractory to medical therapy require a second large-bore IV catheter. If the patient has had a major blood group determination and has a negative indirect Coombs test, type-specific blood may be given without waiting for a complete cross-match. Lactated Ringer's solution or normal saline is generously infused until blood can be replaced. Replacement consists of 3 mL of crystalloid solution per 1 mL of blood lost.

2. A Foley catheter is placed, and urine output is maintained at greater than 30 mL/h.

G. **Surgical management of postpartum hemorrhage**. If medical therapy fails, ligation of the uterine or uteroovarian artery, infundibulopelvic vessels, or hypogastric arteries, or hysterectomy may be indicated.

H. **Management of uterine inversion**
   1. The inverted uterus should be immediately repositioned vaginally. Blood and/or fluids should be administered. If the placenta is still attached, it should not be removed until the uterus has been repositioned.
   2. Uterine relaxation can be achieved with a halogenated anesthetic agent. Terbutaline is also useful for relaxing the uterus.
   3. Following successful uterine repositioning and placental separation, oxytocin (Pitocin) is given to contract the uterus.

References: See page 166.

Acute Endometritis

Acute endometritis is characterized by the presence of microabscesses or neutrophils within the endometrial glands.

I. **Classification of endometritis**
   A. Acute endometritis in the nonobstetric population is usually related to pelvic inflammatory disease (PID) secondary to sexually transmitted infections or gynecologic procedures. Acute endometritis in the obstetric population occurs as a postpartum infection, usually after a labor concluded by cesarean delivery.
   B. Chronic endometritis in the nonobstetric population is due to infections (eg, chlamydia, tuberculosis, and other organisms related to cervicitis and PID), intrauterine foreign bodies (eg, intrauterine device, submucous leiomyoma), or radiation therapy. In the obstetric population, chronic endometritis is associated with retained products of conception after a recent pregnancy.
   C. Symptoms in both acute and chronic endometritis consist of abnormal vaginal bleeding and pelvic pain. However, patients with acute endometritis frequently have fevers in contrast to chronic endometritis.

II. **Postpartum endometritis**
   A. Endometritis in the postpartum period refers to infection of the decidua (ie, pregnancy endometrium), frequently with extension into the myometrium (endomyometritis) and parametrial tissues (parametritis).
   B. The single most important risk factor for postpartum endometritis is route of delivery. The incidence of endometritis after a vaginal birth is less than three percent, but is 5 to 10 times higher after cesarean delivery.
   C. Other proposed risk factors include prolonged labor, prolonged rupture of membranes, multiple vaginal examinations, internal fetal monitoring, maternal diabetes, presence of meconium, and low socioeconomic status.
   D. **Microbiology.** Postpartum endometritis is usually a polymicrobial infection, produced by a mixture of aerobes and anaerobes from the genital tract.

Type and Frequency of Bacterial Isolates in Postpartum Endometritis*	
Isolate	**Frequency (percent)**
Gram positive	
Group B streptococci	8
Enterococci	7
S. epidermidis	9
Lactobacilli	4
Diphtheroids	2
S. Aureus	1
Gram negative	
G. vaginalis	15
E. Coli	6
Enterobacterium spp.	2
P. mirabilis	2
Others	3

Isolate	Frequency (percent)
Anaerobic	
S. bivius	11
Other Bacteroides spp.	9
Peptococci-peptostreptocci	22
Mycoplasma	
U. urealyticum	39
M. hominis	11
C. trachomatis	2

E. Vaginal colonization with group B streptococcus (GBS) is a risk factor for postpartum endometritis; GBS colonized women at delivery have an 80 percent greater likelihood of developing postpartum endometritis.

F. **Clinical manifestations and diagnosis**. Endometritis is characterize, by fever, uterine tenderness, foul lochia, and leukocytosis that develop within five days of delivery. A temperature greater than or equal to 100.4 °F (38 °C) in the absence of other causes of fever, such as pneumonia, wound cellulitis, and urinary tract infection is the most common sign.

G. **Laboratory studies** are not diagnostic since leukocytosis occurs frequently in all postpartum patients. However, a rising neutrophil count associated with elevated numbers of bands is suggestive of infectious disease. Bacteremia occurs in 10 to 20 percent of patients; usually a single organism is identified despite polymicrobial infection. Blood cultures should be obtained in febrile patients following delivery.

H. **Treatment**

1. Postpartum endometritis is treated with broad spectrum parenteral antibiotics including coverage for beta-lactamase producing anaerobes. The standard treatment of clindamycin (900 mg q8h) plus gentamicin (1.5 mg/kg q8h) is safe and effective, with reported cure rates of 90 to 97 percent.

Antibiotic Regimens for Endometritis

Clindamycin (900 mg IV Q 8 hours) plus gentamicin (1.5 mg/kg IV Q 8 hours)
Ampicillin-sulbactam (Unasyn) 3 grams IV Q 6 hours
Ticarcillin-clavulanate (Timentin)3.1 grams IV Q 4 hours
Cefoxitin (Mefoxin) 2 grams IV Q 6 hours
Ceftriaxone (Rocephin) 2 grams IV Q 24 hours plus metronidazole 500 mg PO or IV Q 8 hours*
Levofloxacin (Levaquin) 500 mg IV Q 24 hours plus metronidazole 500 mg PO or IV Q 8 hours*

* Should not be given to breastfeeding mothers
If chlamydia infection is suspected, azithromycin 1 gram PO for one dose should be added to the regimen

---

2. Treatment should continue until the patient is clinically improved and afebrile for 24 to 48 hours. Oral antibiotic therapy is not necessary after successful parenteral treatment, unless bacteremia is present.

3. Modifications in therapy may be necessary if there is no response to the initial antibiotic regimen after 48 to 72 hours. Approximately 20 percent of treatment failures are due to resistant organisms, such as enterococci which are not covered by cephalosporins or clindamycin plus gentamicin. The addition of ampicillin (2 g q4h) to the regimen can improve the response rate. Metronidazole (500 mg PO or IV q8h) may be more effective than clindamycin against Gram negative anaerobes but is generally not used in mothers who will be breastfeeding.

References: See page 166.

Postpartum Fever Workup

History: Postpartum fever is ≥100.4 F (38 degrees C) on 2 occasions >6h apart after the first postpartum day (during the first 10 days postpartum), or ≥101 on the first postpartum day. Dysuria, abdominal pain, distention, breast pain, calf pain.

Predisposing Factors: Cesarean section, prolonged labor, premature rupture of membranes, internal monitors, multiple vaginal exams, meconium, manual placenta extraction, anemia, poor nutrition.

Physical Examination: Temperature, throat, chest, lung exams; breasts, abdomen. Costovertebral angle tenderness, uterine tenderness, phlebitis, calf tenderness; wound exam. Speculum exam.

Differential Diagnosis: UTI, upper respiratory infection, atelectasis, pneumonia, wound infection, mastitis, episiotomy abscess; uterine infection, deep vein thrombosis, pyelonephritis, pelvic abscess.

Labs: CBC, SMA7, blood C&S x 2, catheter UA, C&S. Gonococcus culture, chlamydia; wound C&S, CXR.

References

References may be obtained at www.ccspublishing.com/ccs

Index